If after you've had the first bite of chocolate or ice cream or potato chips or salted nuts or Mexican food or bread or any other food you can name, you can't stop eating, you are a yo-yo dieter. If you shovel food into your mouth when you are upset or angry or things are going badly for you, you are a yo-yo dieter. If you turn to food to keep you going when you are under stress or are tired or anxious or bored, you are a yo-yo dieter. If you are a successful dieter but think just a few more bites of your favorite food won't hurt, you are a yo-yo dieter.

No matter what your downfall is, this book will help you out of the Yo-Yo Syndrome.

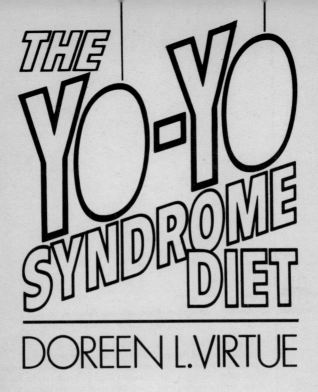

THE YO-YO SYNDROME DIET

DOREEN L. VIRTUE

Harper Paperbacks

Harper & Row, Publishers, New York
Grand Rapids, Philadelphia, St. Louis, San Francisco
London, Singapore, Sydney, Tokyo, Toronto

Harper Paperbacks a division of Harper & Row, Publishers, Inc.
10 East 53rd Street, New York, N.Y. 10022

A hardcover edition of this book was published in 1989 by Harper
& Row, Publishers, Inc.

First Harper Paperbacks printing: February, 1990

Printed in the United States of America

HARPER PAPERBACKS and colophon are trademarks of Harper
& Row, Publishers, Inc.

10 9 8 7 6 5 4 3 2 1

Acknowledgments

ALL of my dealings with the highly professional and personable Harper & Row staff have greatly impressed me, and I want to thank them for their assistance and expertise. My gratitude to Carol Cohen for her skillful editing and suggestions, William Shinker for believing in this project and Susan Randol for her energetic attention to the book's finishing touches and also to Diana Puglisi, Arthur Neuhauser and Eric Wirth for their recommendations during copy-editing and production.

I can't thank my agents, Mel Berger and Irene Webb, enough for all the help and encouragement they've given me. Their guidance and enthusiasm about this book helped make the process of writing it a pleasure. Thank you, also, to their assistants, Kate Edwards and Lauren Karassik Weiss.

Contents

Part Two

Part One

Why Your Weight Goes Up and Down

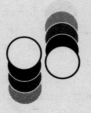

Before starting a diet, check with your doctor to be sure it is appropriate for you to go on a diet and that the diet you have selected is suitable for you.

While following the diet, if you experience any unexpected or unusual reactions or symptoms, consult your doctor promptly.

The case histories in this book are based on actual situations but in some instances the cases are composited, and in all instances the names and all identifying details about each person have been changed.

1

The Yo-Yo Syndrome

GINA, a 42-year-old brunette, tried all the diets and none of them worked for her. "I need to lose thirty pounds, but just keep putting more weight on!" she told me.

Gina was desperate to lose weight. Standing 5 feet 6 inches tall, she weighed 155 pounds. She had been on one diet after another since age 15, and had lost and gained her excess weight too many times to remember. Gina suffered from the Yo-Yo Syndrome; that is, her weight chronically fluctuated up and down.

For people like Gina, losing weight has little to do with dieting. She knew, as so many of us do, that more calories have to be burned than consumed. We've read countless diet books and joined Weight Watchers and other diet clubs; we're *experts* on dieting. Yet, for all this knowledge, we cannot keep the lost weight off! Why? Because the Yo-Yo Syndrome has little to do with the body and a lot to do with the mind. We use food to relax, as a reward or for short-term relief from stress or emotional pain.

Through the special eating plan described in this book, and by pinpointing the issues that kept Gina overweight, I helped her get the weight off. Today, there is no reason to believe that Gina will ever be heavy again.

If you follow the Yo-Yo Syndrome Diet, you, too, *will* lose weight in such a way that you can comfortably keep it off for the rest of your life. Whether you need to lose 5 or 150 pounds, this eating plan will work where diets have failed you.

What Is the Yo-Yo Syndrome?

Up until four years ago, my closet held skirts and pants in sizes 5 through 15—all belonging to me. My weight had fluctuated enough to earn me the name "Skinny" in the 4th grade and "Fatso" in the 6th. This up-and-down pattern continued into adulthood and through the birth of my two children.

My bulging thighs and flabby stomach made me depressed. To feel better, I'd grab a carton of chocolate ice cream or a bag of chocolate-chip cookies. I'd overeat desserts and baked goods until my jeans wouldn't zip up and I couldn't button my skirts. Too-tight clothes would signal me to lose weight again. I'd then go on the latest fad diet until, in utter misery from feeling deprived and half-starved, I'd lose the 15 to 30 extra pounds. Once thin, I'd assume it was okay to resume eating anything I liked and the cycle would begin again.

I was suffering from the Yo-Yo Syndrome, a pattern of losing and gaining weight over and over again. Women are particularly vulnerable, although men certainly suffer from the syndrome, too. All sorts of attempts are made to lose weight. Skipping meals and fasting. Exercising and fad diets. But the weight is just a symptom of the true syndrome, which is a sequence of psychological and physical patterns common to Yo-Yo Syndrome sufferers.

If you have been on many diets in your lifetime but are currently unhappy with your weight, if you tend to binge on a certain type of food (chocolate, potato chips, bread, spicy foods, cheese, etc.), if you eat more when you're angry or stressed, chances are you suffer from the Yo-Yo Syndrome. If so, you know firsthand the frustrations of looking for the magical cure that will take your weight off and keep it off for good.

Most diet books and programs try to deal with the problem on a purely physical basis, promising that if you combine foods in certain ways or eliminate fats, carbohydrates or dairy products, your excess weight will disappear forever. The limited long-term success of these diet plans is clearly illustrated by the way "new" diets are constantly sought after and are propelled into best-selling books, one after another. If any of these books contained *the* secret to permanent weight loss, there would be no need for new diet books.

These books haven't been permanently adopted by many dieters because they don't address the main reasons people break their diets. In fact, most diets contribute to dieters' preoccupation with food by asking them to constantly weigh and measure their food, *thus leading to more preoccupation with food and eating than if they weren't on a diet!* These diets are often a lot of work and are difficult to stay on for more than a few weeks or months. What has been needed is an eating plan that takes one's mind off of food, so it can easily become a lifelong habit. That eating plan is part of the Yo-Yo Syndrome Diet.

Other types of books say it's okay to be overweight. Society is too obsessed with being thin, the authors write, with an underlying message to "stop worrying about your weight so much. You're fine just as you are." While I'm the first to agree that the media have contributed to the national obsession with losing weight, I don't think it's wrong to want to look and feel your best.

Many scientifically sound studies have pointed out that thin, attractive people consistently receive better treatment from strangers, spouses, children, employers and co-workers. Is this fair? Probably not. But is unfairness any reason to ignore such a strong social bias? In truth, we're probably all prejudiced in favor of aesthetic beauty, whether it means appreciating a shapely body, a breathtaking flower, an impressive mansion or a skillfully filmed movie.

There's nothing wrong with wanting to lose weight. It's not superficial—it's realistic! Being thin doesn't erase all of life's problems, but in many ways it does make life easier. When you lose weight permanently, you feel better psychologically and physically. And feeling better makes your life better.

If your weight constantly fluctuates, you are paying dearly for it. Your ever-changing fat levels damage your heart and overall health, your self-esteem and confidence, your relationships with people and your pocketbook.

The reasons why people suffer from the Yo-Yo Syndrome vary and for that reason, there's not one absolute right way for everyone to lose weight. The Yo-Yo Syndrome Diet takes this individuality into account and offers you a way to match your weight-loss program with your unique personality and situation. Here are some typical cases of Yo-Yoers—find which one most reminds you of yourself:

1. *Those Who Can't Stop Eating Certain Foods: "The Binge Eaters."* Becky, who prided herself on always being organized and in control, couldn't understand why she lost self-control and went on a binge every time she ate something with chocolate in it. Similarly, JoAnn found that she couldn't keep a quart of ice cream in her freezer without finishing it off in one sitting. Chocolate, sweets, bread, salty junk foods, ice cream and frozen yogurt, nuts, cheese, creamy salad dressings, and spicy Italian or Mexican dishes are very common binge foods.

2. *Those Who Use Food for Comfort: "The Emotion Eaters."* Janice's high-pressure job put her in many upsetting situations, yet she had difficulty telling people she was irked by their behavior. After work, Janice would have a whole day's worth of anger saved up inside of her, and as soon as she got home each evening she would head right for the refrigerator to feel better.

In addition to being used as a cover-up for anger, food is used to combat feelings such as tiredness. Cindy felt exhausted after a day of chasing her toddler and caring for her newborn baby. To give herself enough energy to prepare dinner each evening, she'd eat sugary snacks such as candy or cookies and wash them down with a cola.

3. *Those Who Use Food to Feel Better About Themselves: "The Self-Esteem Eaters."* Hillary put her husband and kids first and spent what little extra money the family had on them—never on herself. She wore old double-knit pants and ragged shirts, and often forgot to put on makeup. In the ten years of her marriage, Hillary gained over 40 pounds because overeating was another way Hillary mistreated herself.

4. *Those Who Use Food When They're Under Stress: "The Stress Eaters."* Rosalyn, a middle management executive at an insurance company, never felt as if she had enough time to get everything done. "I put in fifty hours a week at work," she says, "then have to come home and take care of my family. My weekends are spent doing laundry and grocery shopping—my only 'fun' seems to be when I eat!"

Unfortunately, Rosalyn's choice of using food as a stress-management tool had resulted in a 30-pound weight gain over the past two years. "Before I took this job, I took a lot of pride in how I looked," Rosalyn explained. "But now, I just don't have any time to exercise or go to a diet club! I've almost resigned myself to the fact that I'm gonna end up being fat like my mother was."

5. *Those Who Gradually Increase Their Food Consumption: "The Snowball Effect Eaters."* Diane had been gaining and losing the same 15 pounds as long as she could remember: "It never fails," she explained, "I'll no sooner get the weight off than I'll start putting it back on again!" On closer examination, we found that Diane would lose weight by cutting the size of her meals. Once the 15 pounds were off, Diane used to stop paying attention to her portions, and her meals would grow larger and larger until all the weight was regained.

Every winter, Darlene, another Snowball Effect Eater, would put on 20 extra pounds. "At least I can hide it under bulky sweaters and coats," she told me, "but it sure would be nice to stay the same weight year-round for once in my life." Each spring would find Darlene vigorously dieting and exercising to prepare for summertime and bathing suit season, a pattern she was extremely tired of.

Recognize Your Yo-Yo Syndrome Style

The Yo-Yo Syndrome Diet involves steps that are thoroughly outlined in this book. The steps aren't particularly difficult, but each one is important. For that reason, don't read ahead of yourself. In other words, complete each step as you read it in this book, and read the steps one at a time. Do the steps in order as you find them and you will lose weight, be able to keep it off forever, and feel good about yourself, emotionally and physically.

It's very important that you understand *why* you overeat as a means of finding out *how* to keep the weight off for good. This book is divided into two parts: in the first, you will pinpoint why you overeat and read about basic ways to overcome these tendencies. In the second half of the book you will find the actual Yo-Yo Syndrome Diet, along with many suggestions for lifestyle shifts and changes that go hand-in-hand with permanent weight loss.

Take a moment now to single out which kind of Yo-Yo Syndrome Dieter you are: "The Binge Eater," "The Emotion Eater," "The Self-Esteem Eater," "The Stress Eater," or "The Snowball Effect Eater."

Some people find they suffer from a combination of Yo-Yo Syndrome styles. If so, then you should pay attention to the Yo-Yo Syndrome Diet steps given for all the styles that apply to you. In fact, most Yo-Yoers are able to see themselves in all five of these styles from time to time. For that reason, it's a good idea to read all the material in this book as you begin your diet.

No matter what type of Yo-Yoer you are, this book will help you out of the Yo-Yo Syndrome. You'll understand why you keep putting the weight back on after losing it, and how you can finally achieve your ideal weight—and maintain it—without yo-yoing.

The weight-loss plan is the product of research derived from several resources. First, my own struggle to overcome the Yo-Yo Syndrome was my painful initiation into the world of endless diets that never quite lived up to their promises. Somehow, that quick weight-loss answer always seemed to evade me.

Second, my work as a psychotherapist treating overweight people has enabled me to see firsthand the patterns of Yo-Yo Syndrome sufferers. I've spent countless hours with frustrated dieters and have learned what they overeat and why. I've also seen the Yo-Yo Syndrome Diet work on clients who were convinced they'd never lose their excess weight.

Third, the information in this book is drawn from the latest research on obesity. There are some vital facts about metabolism and brain chemistry that help explain the Yo-Yo Syndrome. The researchers in this field are tracking some very exciting areas that also clarify why most diets aren't effective.

The Yo-Yo Syndrome Diet has worked for me and for my clients, and it will work for you, too, if you study and use the principles in this book.

2

The Binge Eaters

STYLE NUMBER ONE in the Yo-Yo Syndrome is the Binge Eater. The Binge Eater really doesn't want to overeat, but feels *driven* to do it. Pamela, for example, wanted to stay away from eating sweets more than anything. But invariably when she'd go into the kitchen, she'd think about the cookies in her cupboard.

Pamela struggled to stay away from the cookies, thinking, "No, I won't eat them!" Then she'd think, "Well, just one won't hurt," so she'd head toward the cupboard—and then stop herself with a "No!" Then she'd tell herself, "Yes, I will have one!" The more she fought with herself, the more anxious she'd become. The more anxious she became, the more she wanted a cookie. After a few more minutes of this war inside her, Pamela knew that eating a cookie would calm her down. She grabbed the cookie bag before she had time to talk herself out of it. Chewing away, Pamela sighed with relief.

Pamela's eating was compulsive, because she really didn't want to eat the cookies. It's one thing to willingly choose to eat a cookie, but quite different to struggle with yourself and then feel defeated after giving in to the overpowering urge to eat.

When Audrey's husband complained about her binge eating, Audrey laughed. "I thought he was jealous of the way I could eat anything I wanted," she remembered, "but I hadn't let myself notice that I'd put on thirty-five pounds in two years." Audrey denied her problem with food because she held on to a major misconception about overeating. "I thought binge-eaters were those people who ate everything in sight for three hours and then threw it all up," she said. "I wasn't doing that, so I thought I wasn't binging."

Whenever you eat for reasons other than physical hunger or emotions you are binge eating. You don't have to eat a refrigerator full of food to be on an eating binge. A binge can consist of eating just one cracker if that cracker is compulsively eaten. If you don't really want to eat that cracker but feel anxiously compelled to eat it anyway, then your eating is out of control.

Melanie, a dark-haired, well-groomed 27-year-old secretary, was able to control her eating during breakfast and lunch. But when she got home at 4 o'clock, she'd head straight for the refrigerator and compulsively search for something sweet to eat.

"I'd pull out a carton of ice cream and promise myself

I'd eat just one spoonful," Melanie explained. "But that first one would taste so good, that I always ended up having another. And then another. Sometimes I'd eat half the carton before realizing what I'd done."

Melanie's 4 o'clock binges eventually put 15 extra pounds on her, and she knew she'd have to cut out the sweets in order to successfully lose weight. She was incredibly frustrated by the time she came into our clinic for help with her Yo-Yo Syndrome. "I just can't get by until dinner without overdoing my eating!" she complained.

Melanie was out of control over ice cream—it was her binge food. A binge food is any substance that makes you want to eat more and more food. Every Binge Eater's binge food is different, but it usually is sweets such as chocolate, cookies, candy, ice cream or frozen yogurt; salty junk foods like nuts or potato chips; spicy foods such as Mexican, Italian or Cajun dishes; cheeses and sauces; or baked goods.

Rhonda, for instance, was a late-night Binge Eater whose binge food was potato chips. Every night she'd unwind in front of the television set with a bag of chips and some salsa or dip. Though Rhonda would try to eat just three or four chips, she'd always finish the bag and go on to eat pretzels, crackers or popcorn. Every morning Rhonda would promise herself to stay away from the salty junk foods . . . only to break the promise that evening.

A 38-year-old homemaker, Candace always put off eating her first meal until the kids were off to school.

Then at 10 o'clock it was time for her favorite game show, and Candace would fix buttered english muffins to eat during the hour to come. All too soon, her favorite show would end and Candace would be left with a two-story house to clean. She'd toast more bread instead—crunchy-brown, with pools of butter, that toast comforted Candace when the rest of the day's activities often seemed drab or depressing.

For Melanie, Rhonda and Candace, overeating was triggered when they ate their binge foods. Melanie's ice cream, Rhonda's salty junk foods and Candace's toast had the same effect: they made the women feel better, and that feeling led to wanting more.

Yo-Yo Syndrome Binge Eaters are unable to stop eating once they taste their binge food. Even after months of dieting, and after all the work that went into losing weight, one taste of a binge food destroys their efforts and their weight yo-yoes one more time.

Sometimes craving more of the binge food doesn't occur right away. After losing between 10 and 55 pounds all those countless times, I'd believe I was cured of overeating and gaining weight. So, ignoring my past history of yo-yoing, I'd experiment by eating chocolate ice cream. "Now that I'm thin," I'd rationalize to myself every time, "maybe I'm like those people who can eat anything and not gain weight." So I'd eat a bowl of double chocolate chip and the next day, my scale would show I hadn't gained any weight. I'd then conclude I could eat my binge food without suffering any consequences.

Eating my binge food, though, caused me to crave more chocolate ice cream. So the next day I'd eat two more scoops, and still not gain weight. I paid attention only to my weight and ignored the fact that the second dish of ice cream was eaten compulsively. By the third day, my ice cream eating would be out of control again, and I'd be back on my way to daily overeating. Ice cream, my binge food, has always been my downfall.

If you are a Yo-Yo Syndrome Binge Eater, you may have identified your particular binge food, but to help you really get a clear picture of the scope of this phenomenon, the next section will explore common binge foods.

Step #1 for Binge Eaters:
Identify Your Binge Foods

Some Binge Eaters have no trouble identifying their binge food. They know without a doubt that they can't eat just one cashew or one brownie. Other people say that *all foods* are their binge food and it certainly can seem that way when you overeat at every meal, every day. I've found, though, that Binge Eaters have at least one particular food that triggers an eating binge. If you are a Binge Eater, the first step in your Yo-Yo Syndrome Diet is to identify what your binge food is, for reasons that are discussed later in this chapter. The descriptions below may help you to identify your binge food. While reading them, ask yourself these questions:

- How does eating this food make me feel? Calm or energized, happy or depressed? What other emotions does it trigger in me?
- Have I ever been able to eat just one piece or bite of this food? Do I want more the next day or later that week?
- When I eat this food, do I feel guilty or nervous afterward?
- How many times have I begun an eating binge because I've tasted this food?

CHOCOLATE

"Chocoholic" has found its way into American vocabulary with a tongue-in-cheek connotation attached. For many Binge Eaters, though, chocolate is no laughing matter because of the way it keeps their weight constantly fluctuating. Let's say you decide to diet in time for the holidays. After three or four months of rigorous self-discipline and losing 20 or 30 pounds, you feel really good about the weight loss. Then comes Christmas. And with it, the inevitable boxes of chocolate candy.

Feeling foolish over worrying about "just one chocolate," you reach for the candy box and find you cannot stop with just one piece. You think, "Well I've blown my diet for this day, so I may as well indulge." At that point, an eating binge ensues. It may begin with chocolate and end up with any other type of food that happens to be around.

Recent studies help to explain why some of us crave chocolate: First, chocolate contains powerful stimulants that lead to a sudden surge of energy right after it's eaten. Second, chocolate contains large amounts of a chemical called phenylethylamine, which produces feelings of happiness. This is also the substance produced by your brain when you are feeling romantic love. I've noticed that my clients who are having marital or dating difficulties have stronger cravings for chocolate than they had before the relationship difficulties. Their desire for chocolate is actually a desire for feelings of love. This observation was recently backed up by a study showing that "chocoholics" have higher-than-normal tendencies to fall in love easily and be devastated by romantic rejection. In addition, hormonal fluctuations make many women crave chocolate before and during their menstrual cycles.

Finally, if the other chemicals weren't enough, the *aroma* of chocolate contains another mood-influencing substance called pyrazine. When inhaled, pyrazine activates the pleasure center of the brain, leading to feelings of contentment.

Many chocoholics control their cravings by switching to sugarless chocolate items such as sorbitol, diet chocolate soda or non-fat chocolate frozen yogurt sweetened with honey or fructose. Other people find that when they reduce or eliminate caffeine from their diets, chocolate cravings subside considerably. Other ways to reduce chocolate cravings are discussed in Chapter 7.

OTHER SWEETS

Some Binge Eaters aren't tempted by chocolate at all, but are drawn toward other sugary desserts. Candy, cookies, doughnuts, ice cream, pies, cakes and even soda pop are all difficult for dieters to resist, but if this is your binge food category, staying away from these desserts can seem almost impossible.

Sylvia was a dessert binger who really had a weakness for doughnuts. Every morning, she'd stop by the doughnut shop under the guise of picking up a two-dozen box for her co-workers, but Sylvia would always eat half the box or more herself. When she decided to go on the Yo-Yo Syndrome weight-loss plan, Sylvia had to confront the fact that she was really buying the doughnuts for herself, not to be the nice person at work.

Sugar gives the body a big boost of adrenaline and leads to feelings of euphoria and high energy. The high soon topples, however, leading to a slump in emotion and energy levels. And the cravings for more sugar begin.

Sweet desserts are also loaded with another substance connected with mood regulation: carbohydrates. Carbohydrates activate a brain chemical called seratonin, which produces a calming effect and reduces feelings of depression. It appears that some people are more sensitive to carbohydrate-induced seratonin than others.

One study showed that the same amount of carbohydrates can make some people feel jittery and anxious, while making others feel calm. Sugary desserts such as pie, cookies and cake often contain more carbohydrates than do chocolate-flavored foods, which may explain why some people can leave chocolate alone but can't stay away from other sweets. How you react to carbohydrates depends on your chemical makeup, and since everyone's brain chemical levels are different (as well as everyone's preferences for mood states—some people prefer to be calm while others like to be more energetic), it make sense that everyone's binge foods are different.

Like chocoholics, sugar bingers can control cravings by switching to low-calorie, artificially sweetened versions of their favorite treats. Choose candies, cookies and baked goods sweetened with sorbitol or fructose (but note that these items also can be loaded with calories, and make sure they don't exceed the calorie allowance for snacks outlined in Chapter 8, "Your Eating Plan").

Artificially sweetened diet sodas and chewing gum are also helpful when you crave sugar. And by far one of the best ways of combating dessert cravings is by having something naturally sweetened, such as fresh fruit or raisins.

SALTY JUNK FOODS

Nuts, pretzels and potato chips appeal to Binge Eaters who crave foods that are crunchy and high in fat. People who overeat when they're angry tend to pick crunchy foods on which to take out their aggressions. Christina, for example, was continually upset at her husband for not pitching in around the house. She'd come home from work and find him asleep on the couch while the children ran around the house unsupervised. Usually, she'd console herself by munching on a bowl of buttered popcorn or some potato chips. As she viciously crunched away, her anger toward her husband usually subsided.

In addition, studies now show that overeaters have a "fat tooth" as well as the proverbial sweet tooth. In other words, many overeaters crave fat in the foods that they choose. One reason is that fat stays in the stomach longer than other food properties, leading to a sense of fullness for a greater length of time. Salty junk foods have extremely high fat content, and people whose binge food is in this category have a hard time cutting back because their stomachs are accustomed to holding a certain amount of fat. Because it takes approximately one month to adjust to a low-fat diet, Yo-Yo Syndrome sufferers who attempt to stay away from salty junk foods may feel hungry all the time and thus be tempted to eat "just one" chip, nut or pretzel. But as with the other binge foods, there's no such thing as "just one."

Those who binge on nuts are also attracted to the chemical pyrazine in their aroma. The vapors of pyrazine trigger the pleasure center of the brain, leading to feelings of enjoyment as you smell or eat the nuts. This, of course, also adds to the binge food properties of this food because it's tough to break away from something that makes you feel good. And since chocolate also contains pyrazine, chocolate-covered nuts are a particularly common binge food.

There is also a physiological need to chew a certain number of times every day. If this need isn't satiated— for instance, if you eat only soft or creamy foods—it can lead to cravings for something crunchy to satisfy that urge to chew. You can fulfill that need by chewing carrots, celery, frozen sugar-free pops or sugarless gum.

DAIRY PRODUCTS

While you may turn to crunchy foods because you are angry, cravings for soft dairy products such as cream cheese, ice cream, frozen yogurt, dressings and sour cream often signal a desire for comfort or nurturing. Sandy, a 32-year-old homemaker and mother of three, continually craved buttermilk "ranch-style" salad dressing. Before she went on the Yo-Yo Syndrome Diet eating plan, Sandy poured the dressing on practically everything she ate.

Dairy products do have a satisfying texture to some Yo-Yo Syndrome sufferers, and they also contain a number of chemicals that reduce feelings of depression and lead to feelings of calmness. For instance, dairy products contain high amounts of L-tryptophan. This chemical causes soothing physical and emotional feelings, but in order for L-tryptophan to fully metabolize in the brain and bring on the strongest relaxation effect, carbohydrates must be present with the dairy product.

This chemical combination may explain why many people binge when they eat cheese with crackers, bread or tortillas, as well as other dairy product/carbohydrate mixtures.

Dairy products also contain large quantities of choline, a substance that spurs production of a brain chemical responsible for feelings of happiness and contentment. This binge food category, as with the others, is full of mood-regulating chemicals.

Dairy food bingers can reduce their cravings with this two-part plan: first, have cottage cheese, using the guidelines in Chapter 8, with your breakfast every morning. One cup of low-fat cottage cheese contains almost 350 milligrams (mg) of L-tryptophan; this one cup will satiate your desire for L-tryptophan and reduce your cravings for the rest of the day.

Second, if you binge on cottage cheese, though, or if your cravings tend to occur later in the day, then try taking one 500-mg L-tryptophan tablet one hour before your cravings normally occur. More information on this amino acid appears in Chapter 7.

BREADS AND STARCHES

One thing I've noticed in my years as a psychotherapist is that many people are in occupations involving their binge food. Harold, for instance, couldn't have been in a worse occupation for someone whose binge food was bread: he drove a bakery truck. Imagine that, if you will! Harold's binge food constantly followed him around for nine hours at a time. Not surprisingly, he finally decided that controlling his weight meant leaving the bakery business.

People turn to bread, pasta, rice or potatoes because the high carbohydrate content of these foods increases the brain's serotonin levels. This leads to calm, happy feelings. In addition, the yeast and glucose in breads are both stimulants that provide mood and energy boosts. The boost, however, is soon followed by a drop in blood sugar, causing low energy levels and mild depression. The vicious cycle of overeating bread and other starches begins when Binge Eaters eat more of these foods to feel good again.

Bread is a difficult binge food to contend with, because it's such an intrinsic part of mealtime. Not only is bread served as a side dish at most restaurants, but every kind of meat imaginable is breaded. Pasta, closely related to bread, is also hidden in salads and main dishes.

Bread is definitely hard to avoid. I know, because it is one of my binge foods. I could never stop at one piece of bread, one roll or one serving of a pasta dish. I tried, I *really* tried to control my bread eating. But after at least 20 more experiments in which I attempted to eat just one piece of bread with a meal and failed, I knew I was up against a powerful internal process that wasn't under voluntary control. Like other Binge Eaters, I'd like nothing better than to be able to eat a roll with my dinner. But I can't stop at one.

Most bread bingers are able to curtail their cravings by eating other forms of starch at their meals, such as rice, corn or potatoes. Chapter 8 outlines specific guidelines for controlling your portions of these other starches.

SPICY MEALS

Spicy meals such as Mexican, Italian, Cajun or Szechuan are also common binge foods.

Helena, for example, always knew that Mexican food was the downfall of her diets. Every time she'd lose weight, she'd have to avoid burritos, tacos, and tostadas —not because of the calories in these foods, but because she couldn't stop eating them once she started.

She'd go to a taco stand and promise herself, "I'll just have one." Then, as she stood at the order window, she'd smell the aroma of spicy beef and melting cheese and end up ordering two or three burritos. "I'd be so embarrassed about ordering that much food for myself that I'd order two sodas so the restaurant help wouldn't think it was all for me," Helena remembered.

Mexican and Italian meals that combine aged cheese such as parmesan or cheddar, with yeast-laden tortillas, pizza crust or noodles, and beef or chicken, are loaded with the chemical tyramine. This powerful stimulant leads to mood and physical energy elevations almost immediately after the food containing it is eaten. The boost is readily followed by a low, of course, and the overeater begins craving more food to feel good again.

People who overeat spicy foods often have high thresholds for excitement and crave a lot of stimulation in their lives, relationships and meals. Those attracted to spicy foods also tend to take emotional or physical risks, create crises and generally "live life on the edge" because they crave such a high level of excitement.

Of course, the compulsion to overeat spicy food is also triggered if your binge food—say, cheese or bread —is an ingredient in the meal. In cases such as this, it's not spicy foods that trigger the binge, but the binge food ingredient.

One way spicy food Binge Eaters can control binging behavior is by increasing the sensitivity of their taste buds. To do this, stay away from alcohol, coffee and cigarettes for at least one hour before eating, and save them for after dinner instead. Having water, especially with a lime slice, will help keep your palate cleansed and reduce your desire for highly spiced meals.

HEALTH FOODS

For some, health foods are a binge food category. Although it may be surprising, health foods contain many of the same mood-elevating chemicals as other foods. No food is either good or bad—the important question is whether or not the food triggers a binge in *you*.

Peggy was a highly educated woman who prided her-self on her knowledge about health and nutrition. She collected books on the subject, and did most of her shopping at farmers' markets and health food stores. Her diet consisted of natural food, uncontaminated by pesticides, salt or refined sugar.

But Peggy still suffered from the Yo-Yo Syndrome because she binged on health foods. "They taste so good and make me feel so good, too!" Peggy complained. "I just can't stop eating them!" She'd binge on dates, carob drops and dried fruits. She'd overeat granola bars and raisins.

Upon examination of Peggy's eating habits, we found her binges occurred when she ate foods sweetened with highly concentrated natural forms of sugar. The fructose in dried fruits and the honey in granola bars triggered binges in Peggy.

Health food bingers, like Peggy, are usually binging on natural forms of some of the common binge foods named above. Whether it's refined or natural sugar, no matter if it's chocolate or carob, if a food makes you binge then it's your binge food. Health food bingers need to find patterns in the particular type of food they're overeating. If it's in the dried fruits or granola category, then the section on "Other Sweets" above may offer some clues. If the binges occur in response to raw nuts, read the section on "Salty Junk Foods."

Your unique personality, chemical makeup, experiences with the food, and personal taste preferences will decide which foods you turn to most often. Which foods are your binge foods? For some people, it may be two or three of those mentioned above.

If you're not sure what your binge food is, consider the following:

Do you consistently crave a certain type of food?

When you eat it, do you have overwhelming urges to eat more?

Is it hard for you to stay away from that particular food?

Do you find yourself craving more of the food a day or two after you eat it?

Do you want to eat this food even when you're not upset, and there's no stress in your life?

If you answered "yes" to at least three of these questions, then the food in question is your binge food. If you answered "yes" to only one or two of the questions, the food may not be a binge food, but may still place you at high risk for a binge.

Some people are not able to pinpoint what their binge foods are right away, because they've never really paid attention to their reactions to particular foods. If you're still unsure what your binge food is, then take one or two weeks to carefully study your own eating behavior. The best way to do this is to keep a written log of what you eat and your feelings before and after you eat each food. Admittedly, this requires a lot of work, but it will focus your attention on your reactions to different foods.

If you don't care to keep a food journal, then try to make your meals distraction-free (for instance, don't watch television, read or drive while eating) and eat each different food on your plate one at a time so you'll be able to distinguish how each food makes you feel. Pay close attention to your anxiety levels as you eat each food. How do you feel when you eat the dressing on your salad? Do you want more and feel as if you can't get enough of it? How about your dinner roll or baked potato? How do you feel when you're eating dessert?

Look for patterns in your eating and you'll see what your binge foods are. Of course, others who eat regularly with you may already have a good idea what foods you binge on, so you might want to ask them their opinion on this subject.

The Myth of Controlled Eating of Binge Foods

Katie, a 34-year-old law clerk, lost 35 pounds in six months at our clinic by eating normal portions of ordinary foods and abstaining from her binge food, bread.

Once she'd attained her goal weight, Katie decided to experiment with eating her binge food, just once, to see if anything had changed in the way she reacted to it. After all, Katie was doing *wonderfully* in other areas of her life—maybe now she'd be able to have it all, including her binge food.

At dinnertime, Katie sat with her family and buttered herself a warm wheat roll. As soon as it entered her mouth, though, Katie knew she'd made a big mistake because all the old feelings were triggered. "It was like a big bell went off in my head when I ate that roll," Katie recalled. "I felt like everything in the room but the basket of rolls disappeared, and I wanted to finish them all right then." Binge foods remain triggers for overeating. There's an allergic reaction to the chemicals of the binge food and binging follows the eating of that food. It doesn't matter if you stay away from the binge food for months or years, the food will still trigger a binge.

The way you react to your binge food now is exactly the way you will always react to it. If, on the other hand, you are able to control your eating when you're calm and only binge on the food when you're upset, then you're not Binge Eating, you are instead Emotion Eating (which is described in Chapter 3). Binge Foods, in contrast, remain triggers for binges *even when you're feeling calm, relaxed and at peace with yourself.* I wish there were a cure for Binge Eaters, because I would be the first one to line up at the ice cream counter and the bakery if I truly knew I would be able to stop at just one. Others who miss their binge food feel the same way.

But in the Yo-Yo Syndrome Diet, binges need to be avoided at all costs. They put all the weight back on us after months of working at getting the pounds off. They make us feel bad about ourselves, because after a binge we feel guilty, weak and out of control. One of the best ways to avoid ever binging again is to avoid those foods that are clearly your binge foods.

On the other hand, if you are able to eat *just one* of a certain food, or if you overeat only when you're experiencing a "fattening feeling" (see Chapter 3), then you need not eliminate that food from your diet. In other words, if you can eat one piece of candy, one biscuit, one potato chip or one cookie and not feel compelled to voraciously consume the rest, then you can eat that food and still lose weight. Similarly, if you only binge on these foods when you're upset, then you'll have to avoid those foods only during the times when you're feeling emotional and vulnerable to overeating.

The idea of abstinence from binge foods is discussed in detail in Chapters 7 and 10. If you are a Binge Eater, as you progress through the steps of the Yo-Yo Syndrome Diet, you will become ready to abstain from your binge food. For now, your task involves paying close attention to your reactions to the foods you eat. Notice what foods you binge on and look for any connections your hunger pangs and cravings seem to have with emotions or stressors in your life.

By paying attention to both the mind and the body, the Yo-Yo Syndrome Diet provides the tools you need to achieve permanent weight loss. In Chapter 3, we'll look at Style Number Two in the Yo-Yo Syndrome: The Emotion Eaters.

3

The Emotion Eaters

EMOTION EATERS are often at a loss to explain why the pounds they've lost creep back again and may blame themselves for lack of willpower. But, in truth, it's really a lack of self-awareness that's to blame. A lack of awareness of what it is that drives them to eat so much.

One of the main problems that Emotion Eaters face is that they feel hungry a great deal of the time. Their solution in the past has been to eat every time they felt hungry. Unfortunately, since they were so often hungry this meant they would eat a lot of food and gain a lot of weight in the process.

Step #1 for Emotion Eaters:
Identify Your Fattening Feelings

If you are someone who eats to quell upsetting emotions, it's important, at this point, to start paying attention to your feelings of hunger. What you'll probably discover in doing so is that much of what you've labeled hunger is actually something else—anger, boredom, tiredness, depression, loneliness or some other feeling.

Emotion Eaters must become acutely aware of their motivations for wanting to eat. You need this awareness in order to tell whether your stomach's actually empty or you're upset about something and just want to eat to feel better. First, spend the next week analyzing the feelings you have when you're "hungry." The best way to do this is to keep a journal recording how you feel before, during and after you eat. The journal is a black-and-white way of finding patterns in the emotional reasons why you overeat.

Second, the next time you feel like eating, ask yourself if you could possibly be upset instead of hungry. Emotional hunger usually comes on you very *rapidly* and you go from not feeling hungry at all to suddenly feeling as if you're starving. Physical hunger, in contrast, happens gradually. Don't go to the kitchen automatically when you feel hunger pangs. Instead—and this is important—give yourself a mandatory 15-minute "time out" whenever you think you are hungry. During this 15-minute period, think about the possible emotional connections to your hunger—write down, talk or think about what may have upset you during the day. While this step may seem too simple, too easy to work, please give it a try. Emotion Eaters who try this 15-minute "time out" step all tell me enthusiastically that it *really works!*

Third, if you're upset, begin to take action to solve the source of your discomfort. As difficult as this can be, you'll feel a lot better about yourself if you work on solutions to your upsetting situations instead of eating over them. Once you begin to recognize the difference between the emotions that make you want to eat, and actual feelings of hunger, you won't be as apt to reach for food for solutions.

Listed on the following pages are the 16 feelings that Emotion Eaters most often confuse with hunger. Be as honest as you can with yourself in reading this list, because self-awareness is a key ingredient to long-term recovery from the Yo-Yo Syndrome.

1. Anger. Anger is cited in more cases of overeating than any other emotion. Anger, especially when it's repressed, feels very uncomfortable and this discomfort is often confused with hunger. But what feels like hunger is actually a desire to use food to *cover up or mask* the painful emotion, anger.

Women, in particular, have difficulty expressing anger because of societal pressures ranging from parental teachings ("Young ladies shouldn't get angry!") to corporate gameplaying rules ("You'll get ahead in this company if you just smile and agree with management instead of arguing about their policies."). With all this pressure, people sometimes wish they never felt angry—a futile wish, of course, since everyone gets angry at times. People run into trouble with their anger when they ignore their feelings of anger, or pretend they don't exist; or don't express their anger, hoping the feelings will subside if they're ignored long enough; or turn to food in order to feel better.

Barbara did all three when she was angry, and none of them made her feel any better. For the first two months of her Yo-Yo Syndrome Diet, Barbara would come into her weekly counseling session and cry about her overeating and excess weight. It was always apparent from Barbara's tightened fists, her tense, shrill voice and her quick, self-conscious movements that the 37-year-old beautician was quite angry. And this is why she overate.

After listening to her talk, I'd say something to Barbara like, "How were you feeling right before you ate the cake?"

"Oh, I don't know," she'd answer. "Okay, I guess . . . well, maybe just a little upset, too."

"Were you angry at all?"

"No! Of course not. Why would I be angry?"

"Well," I'd reply, "just suppose you were angry, what would you be angry about?"

Barbara eventually realized that she was angry over someone's thoughtlessness—some instance in which Barbara felt victimized but unable to defend herself. She'd be very angry at the perpetrator, usually her husband, boss or mother, but felt she couldn't express her anger. Barbara always told me that "it wouldn't do any good" to tell the other person her feelings. Frustrated and angry, Barbara would turn instead to eating cake and doughnuts to block awareness of her uncomfortable emotions.

Barbara learned how to deal with anger so that her cravings for pastries would subside. She learned that anger is normal and natural, and that no one would reject her for *assertively*—not aggressively—expressing her feelings. Barbara also discovered that it didn't matter whether expressing her feelings resulted in a change in the perpetrator's behavior. What mattered was getting the anger out of her system so that she wouldn't eat over it later. After several months of practicing assertiveness, Barbara began to spontaneously express her feelings to others. She also lost 15 pounds in two months.

2. Fatigue. If anger is the number one psychological reason why people overeat, fatigue is definitely number two. That's why I call it "fat-igue." Late-night overeaters often use food in a vain attempt to energize themselves when they are tired. Shift workers, those who stay up late at night and "workaholics" are especially prone to overeating when fatigued.

There are two ways to break this habit. One is to recognize fatigue in yourself when it occurs. Learn to recognize how it feels when you are emotionally drained or intellectually overstimulated. Once you can label these feelings as fatigue, you won't be as likely to confuse them with hunger.

Second, remember that when you're tired only rest will make you feel better. Food may give you a temporary surge in blood sugar that is reminiscent of feeling rested, but the key word is that the respite is *temporary*. What's more, an eating binge can lead to sluggish, tired feelings the next day as your body tries to break down the high levels of sugar, fat and carbo-hydrates from the binge foods. Rest and regular exercise are the best ways to combat feelings of fatigue. Food only makes things worse!

3. Depression. When life looks grey and gloomy, most Emotion Eaters start to think of ways to feel bet-ter, and their solution to depression usually involves food. People who eat when they're depressed often turn to dairy products such as ice cream (particularly choco-late) and cheese. As precisely as a well-trained pharma-cist, but intuitively, the overeater picks food that alleviates depression; after all, the chemical makeup of dairy products has a neurological effect similar to anti-depressant medications.

Thoughts about cheese melted on pizza or tortillas crept into Martha's mind almost every day as she strug-gled to keep up with her children and still manage to complete her house work. Between the cheddar on her daily omelette and the melted monterey jack or mozza-rella on her lunch and dinner menus, Martha would consume nearly a pound of cheese per day.

It didn't take long to discover that Martha's fattening feeling was depression. She felt discouraged and de-feated, it turned out, because she had dropped out of college after her marriage, giving up her dream of an acting career.

Married to a trucking business owner who regularly worked 12-hour days, Martha saw her role in life as

being little more than an unpaid housekeeper. She was
angry at her husband and resented her kids, but at the
same time felt guilty for harboring these feelings. So
she held them inside and turned the anger inward, at
herself. The result was depression and a *big* appetite for
food.

Once Martha was able to see that she was allowing
herself to be a victim—no one was forcing her to be a
housewife, after all—she returned to college and re-
sumed work on her dream. By restructuring her life to
suit her desires and by following the Yo-Yo Syndrome
Diet, Martha was able to lose 25 pounds and look forward to her future!

Depression occurs for a number of reasons. It can be
traced to:

- Holding in anger (as Martha did).
- A loss, such as losing a job, getting a divorce,
  selling a house, becoming ill or losing a loved one
  (including pets).
- Physical exhaustion or poor nutrition. This type
  of depression, fortunately, is temporary and
  readily responds to rest and a healthy diet.
- "Kicking yourself" and focusing on real or
  imagined negative characteristics in yourself. Try
  to keep your attention focused on your positive
  qualities and remember that everyone makes
  mistakes.
- Feeling like a helpless victim, and seeing the future
  as hopeless. You're not a victim and the future

will be as pleasant or as painful as you set out to make it! You really do create your own life to a large extent.

If you tend to overeat because of depression, first take steps to recognize the source of your sadness. After identifying *why* you feel depressed, work on changing your outlook or your situation. This can happen, of course, through therapy, assertiveness training, or working on the self-esteem exercises in this book. The amino acids discussed in Chapter 7, especially L-tryptophan, also help to combat depression and reduce cravings for dairy products.

4. Loneliness. Even though Donald worked in a huge hospital employing hundreds of workers, he felt very alone. Assuming he could trust no one, Donald rarely revealed anything of a personal nature to his co-workers. Donald, an Emotion Eater, turned to food when he felt lonely: baked goods and nuts such as cashews, peanuts and sunflower seeds, and peanut butter sandwiches. These high-fat bulky foods seemed to fill the void in Donald's life—for a few moments. But the more he'd eat and the more weight he'd gain, the more alienated from others he'd feel.

When Donald first entered therapy, he was convinced that others didn't like him because he was overweight. Donald couldn't have been more wrong. He had to face the fact that it was *Donald* who didn't like Donald, and that he pushed others away from him. Food and fat were just symptoms to cover up his underlying feelings of being unloved and lonely. Once Donald learned to love and accept himself, and began to trust other people, his appetite for peanut butter sandwiches decreased.

Those who eat out of loneliness usually must push themselves to meet new people, even when the prospect seems frightening. Some of the easiest ways to get out and become active with others involve engaging in some sort of organized group activity, such as joining a volleyball team, enrolling in any sort of class or becoming a member of a community club.

5. Insecurity/Inadequacy. At my first counseling position, I felt inadequate a great deal of the time. I worked in a large inpatient alcoholism hospital and we were terribly understaffed. There was always a crisis of some sort with a patient or staff member, and there wasn't much any of us counselors could do to keep the atmosphere positive. Consistently, there was an air of gloom and despair hanging over us. And always, at the end of the day, I was left with feelings of inadequacy that I just hadn't done enough to help the alcoholics and drug addicts in our facility. I'd feel empty and insecure, and I'd want to eat as a result.

Feeling not good enough is an empty sensation. The insecurity and inadequacy that come with self-doubt can feel like a big, black empty hole right in the middle of your gut. It feels uneasy. It doesn't feel good. I think that these feelings are among the toughest to contend with because most of us don't even want to admit we're experiencing them. I know that, at times, I used to believe I was the only person in the world who felt inadequate. And I used to be afraid if I admitted these feelings—even to myself—that it might be true that I *was* inadequate. So I hid the feelings from myself and others, and tried to fill the empty hole with food.

Inadequacy is a very normal feeling! Everyone, including Ph.D.s, M.D.s, rich folks and other successful people, wrestles with self-doubt and feels like a failure at times. Problems with this feeling arise when Emotion Eaters try to ignore or cover up the sense of inadequacy with food, instead of allowing the feeling to run its course or take steps (like returning to college, asking for a raise, etc.) to reduce the reasons for the feeling.

6. Guilt/Responsibility. Kim, a divorced mother of two, was unemployed and worried about meeting next month's expenses. She was also feeling that she'd let her family down because the children needed new school clothes and Kim couldn't afford any. Kim's gnawing conscience and guilt led her to overeat macaroni and cheese and other pasta dishes.

Another patient of mine, Tisha, felt guilty because of her extramarital affair. When she first became involved with her lover, Tisha didn't think that sneaking around to hotel rooms would bother her. But four months into the affair, Tisha began to eat chocolate nonstop as her guilt from the infidelity mounted.

Eating, of course, doesn't resolve the guilt-producing situation. Both Kim and Tisha had to take action at the root of their problems in order to alleviate their guilt. For Kim, this meant cutting down on expenses such as long-distance calls and clothes so she'd have enough money to provide for her children until she could find work. Tisha felt a lot of relief when she broke up with her lover and brought her husband in for marriage counseling.

Besides taking steps to solve the problem, the realization that you are not completely responsible for others, and that you truly can't control anyone else's actions or feelings can also free you of unnecessary guilt. This doesn't mean you should be selfish or thoughtless; just that you should let go of the erroneous notion that you're entirely responsible for the happiness of those around you. No one person is that powerful! Give others credit for the direction they choose to take in their lives.

7. Jealousy. Julia was jealous that her ex-boyfriend, Bob, was dating another woman. She imagined the couple dining and dancing in elegant restaurants, and she tortured herself with fantasies of Bob buying his new girlfriend extravagant and romantic gifts. Though he had been quite *unromantic* and unimaginative when Julia was dating him, she was sure Bob would be the perfect lover with his new girlfriend. And Julia was sure this other woman was prettier, skinnier, smarter and sexier than she herself could ever hope to be. This obsessive jealousy led Julia to nervously snack on cream-filled chocolate cookies, one after another. She'd pace and eat, eat and pace some more.

To break this cycle, Julia's Yo-Yo Syndrome Diet included having her face the fact that Bob was now dating another woman. Julia also came to terms with realizing that Bob was probably just as unromantic with his new girlfriend as he had been with her. And, most importantly, she learned to stop putting herself down and comparing herself to others.

Many "jealousy eaters" I've treated tend to compare themselves unfavorably to others in a process I call "comparing your insides with other people's outsides." This happens whenever you look at other people who *appear* to be so together, happy and confident, and compare this with how you *feel* on the inside. You may become jealous if you assume someone else's life is much better than your own because on the outside he or she appears happier than you. Remember that outside appearances can be deceiving and that to other people, you too, probably appear to have it "all together."

8. Happiness. Kelly was a "happy" overeater. After a year of financial problems and family illnesses, she was relieved when things finally started to go her way. Within two months Kelly got a raise, her mother's cancer went into remission and she finally sold her condominium. Kelly was ecstatic . . . until she found she'd gained 20 pounds in those two months. When Kelly came into my office, her eating was completely out of control and her newfound happiness was in a precarious state.

"Happy" overeaters like Kelly seem to turn to food for two reasons. The first is that when things are going well, they feel very, very good and they want to binge on good feelings. Because the "happy overeater" enjoys food, she wants to eat as much as possible in order to fill up on good feelings. She sees happiness as a limited resource that will run out quickly and needs to be gobbled up before it disappears.

Second, people with low self-esteem often feel they don't deserve happiness or success. So, as soon as aspects of their lives—such as weight loss—start to turn out right, they unconsciously start to sabotage their own success.

Happiness, if you've never had much of it, can seem scary because of its novelty. Even though it seems illogical to wish unhappiness on yourself, some people are uncomfortable with anything but morose, depressing days. They almost *need* a problem or crisis in their life to give them a sense of purpose. This is also an offshoot of Yo-Yo Syndrome Style Number Three, the Self-Esteem Eater, which is discussed further in the next chapter.

If you're a "happy" overeater, it's important to remember that it really is okay to be happy and experience success! In addition, the happiness won't go away or be yanked out of your hands, so *relax*. And most importantly, don't eat over your happiness.

9. Anxiety/Nervousness. Robin would overeat every time she was about to close a real estate deal. Brent found himself stuffing his mouth with food whenever he thought about asking a new girl out for a date. Heather ate bags of sunflower seeds before her midterms and final examinations. Teresa felt as if she was starving when she learned she would have to appear on TV to promote her company's new product line.

Anxiety and nervousness lead to a particular type of overeating—the "picking" variety. This style of eating disguises the amount of food one is eating because only a tiny amount is eaten, bit by bit. But since the eating is continuous, large amounts of food are consumed before the Yo-Yo Syndrome sufferer even realizes what has happened. As if in a blackout or trance, the overeater seeks pacification from anxiety through food.

Those who overeat because of anxiety and nervousness use food to relax, so they need to find alternative methods to unwind. Since anxiety eating is closely related to Stress Eating, people who eat over this fattening feeling would benefit from following Step #1 for Stress Eaters, which is discussed in Chapter 5.

10. Disappointment/Hurt. Elise felt hurt by the way her mother constantly criticized her. Almost daily her mother would call and complain about Elise's choice of husband, job and about how much weight Elise was gaining. In fact, Elise's mother always had something to say about Elise's body when she was growing up. These criticisms hurt Elise's feelings, and she regularly vowed to improve herself so her mom would finally be proud of her. But it seemed there was no pleasing her mother, and the more hurt Elise felt, the more she turned to food to feel better. The more she ate, the more weight she gained. And in this vicious cycle, the more Elise weighed, the more her mother pushed her to lose weight.

Similarly, people often overeat in the face of disappointment. Perhaps a friend lets you down or betrays you. Maybe you didn't get that raise or promotion at work. Or perhaps you feel let down every time you don't win the state lottery. Regardless of its source, disappointment can make you feel alone and hopeless about the future. It can make you lose interest in yourself, make you not care what you weigh or what your body looks like. When you don't care, it's hard to stay away from food.

At times like that, when you feel as if the whole world's against you, it's vital that you stick to the Yo-Yo Syndrome Diet. By staying on the program, you're able to feel good about yourself and that way, at least *one* person's on your side: you!

11. Emptiness/Hollowness. Terry had always let life dictate her choices for her. She went to a local trade school right out of college because she happened to read a newspaper ad for it. After graduation, she accepted the first job offer she received. Even though Terry didn't particularly like her new job—she didn't care for her new location, either—at least it was secure. To Terry, what mattered most was safety and security. But now that she had these qualities in her life, why did she feel so hollow inside? Why did she overeat cake, pastries or doughnuts every night?

Terry felt her life lacked meaning or purpose. My patients who, like Terry, have no sense of where their lives are going, all wrestle with discontentment, emptiness and chronic anxiety. And these feelings all have the same source: settling for unsatisfying positions and not fulfilling one's "mission" in life.

I believe we all have drives or ambitions to do certain things with our lives, and that we owe it to ourselves to try to fulfill those desires. We may not always succeed, but it's very important to at least try. Until we take steps toward our dreams and goals, an upsetting uneasiness lives inside of us. The goal could be anything from getting a high school diploma to graduating from medical school. Writing that novel. Or volunteering at that convalescent hospital. Whatever your personal dream, go capture it! Break the big goal down into smaller, more accessible goals and then take one small step today to bring yourself closer to the life you want to lead. You'll be glad you did.

12. Grief. To find out if unfinished grief could be at the heart of your Yo-Yo Syndrome, ask yourself if thoughts about your losses bring about any of the following:

- A heavy or pressured feeling in your chest?
- Tears to your eyes?
- The desire to think about something else right away?
- Anger or depression?

If you answer "yes" to any of these, you probably have some unfinished griefwork to complete. Though not a pleasant task, spending some time focusing your thoughts on the pain of your loss (preferably with a therapist) could be the key to releasing you from your desire to overeat.

The most remarkable case I ever saw of unfinished griefwork in a Yo-Yo Syndrome sufferer was my patient, Sally. Sally was a very pretty green-eyed brunette, but her 230 pounds were unhealthy for her 5-foot 4-inch stature. Sally had gained over 100 pounds since witnessing her father's death when Sally was a teenager. Instead of grieving over her father's drowning, Sally stuffed herself on high-fat items such as steak, buttered potatoes and salty junk foods.

Our therapy consisted of reading letters that Sally's father had written her and allowing Sally to simply cry, week after week during our sessions, over the fact that her father had died. Once Sally completed her grief-work, her excess weight came off at a rapid and steady rate. By the time Sally was able to read one of her father's letters and not shed tears, she had lost most of the weight and was no longer overeating.

13. Procrastination. Eating is, if nothing else, a very good time-waster. It makes a wonderful excuse for putting off doing an unpleasant task. Ellen, for example, noticed that when she was ready to leave for job interviews, she'd suddenly get insatiably hungry. Her eating usually made her late for appointments with prospective employers, and as a result she'd avoid getting a job offer. The thought of going to work—and possibly being ridiculed, appearing stupid or being fired—terrified Ellen. It was easier to stay home and eat.

Do you ever use food as an excuse to avoid doing some dreaded task? Do you use food to avoid making that phone call or writing that letter? To avoid doing a boring and mundane chore? To avoid completing a complicated or difficult task?

If you have answered "yes" to any of these questions, you've probably already recognized the futility of eating in order to procrastinate. No matter how much food you eat, after all, the task will still remain on your "to do" list. By eating before you tackle the chore, you only make things worse. It makes you feel out of control, fat, sloppy and angry at yourself for eating. And you still have to face the dreaded situation.

Doesn't it make more sense instead to get the task over with (maybe even figuring out a way to enjoy it, too) or delegate the task to someone else or decide that you don't really need to do the chore after all?

14. Fear. Fear often triggers nervous behavior, especially continuous snacking. As if needing some way to displace his pent-up energy, Ted spent the week before his knee surgery emptying the contents of his refrigerator and pantry. He was terrified of the impending surgery and general anesthesia, and worried that something would happen while he was unconscious. It was difficult for Ted to talk about his fears with others because he didn't want to appear weak. But underneath he was afraid. Very afraid. And his method for living with himself for that horribly long week before surgery was to eat as much as he could.

Andrea was also a "fear" overeater, but for Andrea the fear was something she lived with constantly. Ever since she had been beaten and raped three years earlier, Andrea had felt jumpy and afraid that it would happen again. As a result, she overate snack foods. She munched all day long on candy, trail mix, nuts or pretzels—anything that was small and easy to pop into her mouth. The action of chewing on food helped her to feel less nervous and afraid somehow, but it also resulted in her gaining 40 pounds over those three years.

If you're a "fear" eater, it will help for you to examine what it is that you are afraid of. Admitting your

fears will not make them come true; it will make them
have less power over you. And it will also reduce your
desire to overeat!

15. Boredom. Time weighed heavily on Margaret
each day. A 57-year-old grandmother of four, Margaret
never had enough to keep her busy since her husband
had passed away. So she spent her time baking cookies,
cakes and pies "just in case" company dropped by. But
visitors rarely came, and Margaret would end up eating
the desserts herself because she hated to waste food.
When Margaret was finally able to admit that she actually baked the food for herself—not for her hypothet-
ical company—she was forced to find other activities to
fill her time with.

Like people who eat out of procrastination, "boredom bingers" can fill up days, hours, months and years
a bite at a time. They're often anxious with unstructured time and are constantly searching for something
to do. They feel guilty if they're not engaged in some
activity . . . even if it's eating.

If this description reminds you of yourself, it's important to come to terms with underlying issues. Why
isn't it okay to just do nothing once in a while? Do you
always have to be productive to feel good about yourself? Are you trying to please someone or get their approval by staying busy? What other activity would you
like to be engaged in besides eating? Why aren't you
doing that other activity now?

16. Embarrassment. Colleen's husband, Larry, was
an alcoholic who got quite obnoxious when he drank.
He'd invariably embarrass Colleen when they were in

public together by making crude remarks about her. "I just want to disappear when Larry starts saying those awful things!" Colleen cried. Instead of confronting Larry about his behavior and alcoholism, Colleen would stuff her feelings of embarrassment and hurt with food. She'd eat huge portions at restaurants and at parties she'd stand next to the snack table all evening, as if for protection.

Since a big part of Colleen's Yo-Yo Syndrome involved her co-alcoholism (the emotional pain of having a loved one who's an alcoholic), her recovery necessitated involvement in a support group called Al-Anon. This group, similar to Alcoholics Anonymous, is designed specifically to help family members cope with alcoholism. She learned how to be assertive with Larry, and she also discovered his drinking was not her fault. "He had me convinced that he drank because I was fat," she said later. "Now I know that was just an excuse. What a relief!"

Overeating because of embarrassment or self-consciousness often occurs because of unrealistic expectations that you should be perfect. Then, if you do make a mistake—a social blunder or a business error, for instance—you feel as if the world's going to fall apart.

At this point in your Yo-Yo Syndrome Diet, you may notice an increasing awareness of your eating behavior. You may be, by now, almost painfully aware that you don't eat because you are physically hungry. You eat because of emotional hunger. Understanding the reasons for overeating is an important step for Emotion Eaters. By becoming aware of the differences between hunger and uncomfortable emotions, your cravings will diminish.

And remember to keep the 15-minute rule in mind at all times: the minute your mind veers toward thoughts of food and eating, note what time it is. For the next 15 minutes, don't go anywhere near food. Instead, think about what emotions might be triggering your hunger and see if you can work them out in ways not involving food.

One of the best ways to both identify and reduce fattening feelings is to write them down in a private "Feelings Journal." This is one of the best tools for dealing with emotions I've ever used. In fact, a recent study reported its usefulness by concluding that Feelings Journals were almost as effective as therapy in untangling and providing a release for troublesome feelings.

A Feelings Journal consists of a notebook that you carry around for those moments when you feel upset, confused or emotional. At those times, go to a private location such as an office, bathroom or bedroom and write whatever thoughts first come to mind. Then go on writing from there.

Even if you absolutely detest writing, try this exercise just once because I think you'll be pleasantly surprised how much it helps. Remember, this is your private journal and no one has the right to look at it unless you want them to. It's also not an English assignment, so don't worry about spelling, neatness, grammar or punctuation. The only requirement for a Feelings Journal is that you write what you honestly feel.

More suggestions on breaking out of Emotion Eating appear throughout the rest of this book. In the next chapter, we'll look at Yo-Yo Syndrome sufferers who overeat because they lack confidence and security in themselves—the Self-Esteem Eaters.

4

The Self-Esteem Eaters

S TYLE NUMBER THREE in the Yo-Yo Syndrome is the Self-Esteem Eater. Self-Esteem Eaters are those who don't feel very good about themselves and overeat because of it. They lack confidence to leave unfulfilling jobs or unhappy marriages and are afraid to pursue their secret dreams and desires. The vicious cycle takes over when they overeat because they don't like or care about themselves. This leads to weight gains, and subsequently to lower self-esteem, which means even more eating.

Although she was a capable, competent accountant, Robin didn't feel good about herself as a person. The daughter of a depressed, unhappy mother, Robin was constantly told while growing up, "You'll never be pretty! Forget about getting a husband because you're too fat and plain looking." Robin never doubted her mother's disparaging statements, and the 32-year-old blue-eyed, brown-haired woman truly believed she was ugly and stupid.

Evenings and weekends, Robin nibbled constantly, but she never thought of herself as an overeater. In fact, sometimes she wondered how she could eat so little and still be 30 pounds overweight. Robin was unaware of just how much she was eating, a nibble at a time. She was also completely unaware of *why* she was continuously eating: to anesthetize her uneasy feelings about herself.

Another client of mine, Lonnie, was also a Self-Esteem Eater. Painfully shy, Lonnie didn't have any close friends because she was afraid to approach people or to start conversations with co-workers. She lived alone with a house cat and spent her free time holed up in her apartment with a book and a steady supply of snacks and meals.

When I first met Lonnie, she told me she believed others disliked her. "Nobody ever calls or comes over," she complained. Lonnie talked at length about how her "lousy personality" was to blame for her lack of friends. On and on, Lonnie expounded negatively about herself until it was clear that *she,* herself, was the one who disliked Lonnie. And because she didn't like herself, Lonnie would be mean to herself by overeating and staying overweight. Lonnie, in other words, was punishing Lonnie.

Jane, too, was a Self-Esteem Eater. A secretary for a

law firm, Jane had a difficult time standing up for her rights with her boss and co-workers. She often worked overtime without pay because she was afraid to tell her employer "no." She did favors for others, even when she was exhausted and would have preferred to say "I can't."

Jane was a doormat for the people around her because she didn't feel she had the right, or the courage, to assert herself. She soothed her wounded pride at the end of each day with a huge dinner and rich dessert, a practice which kept Jane 20 pounds heavier than she cared to be.

Breaking the destructive cycle of Self-Esteem Eating is tough because it means pulling yourself up by your bootstraps before you feel ready. Let me explain:

Think for a moment about the people in your life whom you like the most, the ones you'd most want to spend time with (not romantic attractions necessarily, though). Most likely, the person you come up with is someone who treats you nicely and who makes you feel good. Someone who you feel really likes you. Who says nice things to you, and who treats you unexpectedly well.

We all like people who are nice to us.

So what happens to us when we don't treat ourselves nicely? How do we feel about ourselves as people when we're inconsiderate to ourselves? When we allow others to walk on us or take advantage of us? The answer, of course, is that we don't like ourselves very much, just as we don't like *anyone* who mistreats us.

The ramification of this, as mentioned a moment ago, is that Yo-Yo Syndrome sufferers whose self-esteem is low don't feel they deserve to be treated nicely. Although I spend a great deal of time helping Self-Esteem Eaters increase their self-esteem level, I usually first have to help new clients feel they deserve to treat themselves well. Because they're so accustomed to kicking themselves and letting everybody else kick them too, they don't know how to stop the cycle.

The paradox of all this is important to understand: before your self-esteem can increase, you must begin to treat yourself as well as you possibly can. This means you must begin taking good care of yourself *before* you feel ready to. You must be nice to yourself even though it feels selfish or makes you feel guilty. Then, *after* a month or two of treating yourself so considerately, your self-esteem will begin to catch up with your new behavior. You'll start to believe you deserve good treatment. Your self-esteem will be much higher at that point.

The section below lists several ways to increase your self-esteem and begin treating yourself better. For the Self-Esteem Eater, this step is as important as the Diet (in Part Two of this book) in order to lose weight and keep it off.

Step #1 for Self-Esteem Eaters: Learning to Love Yourself

You really can like yourself before you've lost your excess weight. In fact, you need to if you're ever going to lose the weight permanently! And it's especially vital if you're ever going to allow yourself to enjoy the fruits of all your hard labor: a trim, attractive body that you, yourself, can appreciate.

Studies show that you need plenty of confidence in yourself in order to successfully lose weight. This is because you need to trust that you'll stick with an eating or exercise plan; without this belief you'll end up saying, "What's the use?" and give up. Unless you like yourself, it's almost impossible to have any confidence in yourself.

If you haven't been good to yourself in a while, it's best to start with basic steps. The self-esteem exercises below are divided into two sections to be completed one at a time. I suggest that you spend at least two weeks on the first section and a month on the second. Of course, taking good care of yourself isn't something that's just temporary; it's an endeavor you'll want to undertake for the rest of your life.

SECTION 1

This section begins with basic exercises that may feel like superficial indulgences at first. Believe me, they're far from trivial—they're designed to set the stage for learning how to be good to yourself. While doing these exercises, you may feel guilty or foolish at first. If you do, don't try to stuff or ignore these feelings, but don't let the feelings stop you from performing each exercise. Each step is important, so don't skip any of them—

even though it may be tempting to do so. Remember that in return for your efforts you'll get what you've always wanted: happiness, self-love and a slim body. Does that sound impossible? If it does, then you really need these exercises badly!

Don't make the mistake of waiting until you're in the mood before beginning these steps—you'll never be in the mood until you take these steps and start to feel better about yourself. In other words, higher self-esteem follows the behavior; first you act "as if" you like yourself, then the actual liking of yourself follows. Start the following steps today.

1. Replace Your Old Clothes

Throw away or donate all your ugly clothes, including pajamas. Even if you were planning to wait until you were at that ideal weight before going clothes shopping, buy yourself some attractive new clothes *this week*. Buy the best, most attractive clothes you can afford. Remember, you deserve them now! By putting off treating yourself well, you virtually guarantee that weight loss won't occur.

As you lose weight on the Yo-Yo Syndrome Diet, get rid of your too-big clothes as you go along. Then buy yourself more new clothes as you shrink out of each new size. Remember that by donating the clothes, you'll have a tax deduction and you'll be helping people less fortunate than yourself. (Remember that the domestic violence shelters can always use donated clothing!)

You won't be wasting money by buying new clothes on your way down the weight scale. Just think about all the money you used to spend on huge meals, snacks, diet clubs, diet doctors and health problems related to your weight. Compared to all that money, these self-esteem steps won't cost all that much. And they'll give you the best return on your money you've ever had!

Looking good now will help raise your self-confidence, make you feel better about yourself, and also garner positive feedback from others. All this will make it much easier for you to lose weight because you'll begin to get in the habit of taking better care of yourself —a habit that will naturally lead you to select foods that are good for you, and to stop stuffing yourself with food beyond the point of satiation. We naturally treat people we like with respect, and this will hold true with your own self, too, as you take better care of yourself.

Along with going to the trouble and expense of dressing well on your "weigh down" the scale, also remember to pay attention to your hair, skin care, makeup, teeth, fingernails and other aspects of personal grooming and hygiene. If you need to see a dermatologist, makeup consultant, dentist, manicurist, speech therapist or other professional, make an appointment right away. Again, the cost will prove to be well worth it . . . think of it as an investment that will return multiple dividends.

2. Treat Yourself Special

Who would be the most special guest you could think of entertaining at your house? Would it be the president or first lady? A movie star? What would you run out and buy, or what would you do differently, if you got a phone call right now telling you that this person was coming to your house for the weekend?

Well, guess what? You're just as special. In fact, you're even more special, because you live with yourself every day and not with the person you first thought about. Since you're so special, you deserve special treatment. Unfortunately, most Self-Esteem Eaters think in terms of settling for second or third best all the time. They do and buy for everyone but themselves, and then they wonder why they don't feel very good about themselves.

Stop settling for a second-rate life! If you'd do something special for someone else, then you can do it for yourself. If you could've afforded it for the president's wife, then you can afford it for yourself. But, you don't have to spend a lot of money to treat yourself well.

- Get out your best china and crystal and put away your plastic cups and stoneware dishes. You deserve to be served on the finest dinnerware, and you'll feel special drinking your water out of elegant stemware.
- Use the full-service pump the next time you go to the gas station. The dollar or so extra won't make that much difference in your budget, but the feeling

of being special will make a big difference in the way you feel about yourself. This ultimately affects your weight, and we don't need to discuss how much money that's cost you, do we?

- Stop going to the bargain table every time you go shopping for shoes or clothes (you do buy yourself new outfits, don't you?). While I'm the first to admit that getting a great bargain can make you feel wonderful, it's also important to buy something that's not on sale once in a while too, if you really want it.

- Treat yourself to a pedicure or a manicure (men, too!).

- Take a luxurious bubble bath, complete with lit candles all around you and a crystal glass full of wine or diet soda.

- Keep a bouquet of fresh flowers in your house at all times. Just put it right on your grocery shopping list instead of the fattening foods you used to buy.

- Buy new underwear. Believe it or not, the quality of your undergarments influences the way you feel about yourself, too. Make sure you ladies have an adequate supply of pretty, well-fitting lingerie and underwear, and men, you deserve to have comfortable and attractive socks and briefs.

- Go away for a mini-vacation all by yourself now and then. This could mean checking into a hotel for the weekend, or house-sitting for a friend who's out of town. Go on a long drive by yourself to your favorite places, even if you say you don't like to be by yourself (as your self-esteem rises, you'll be more comfortable in your own company).

You decide what you want! You don't need anyone's permission to do something that's going to benefit you. Remember that your spouse and children will ultimately be better off, too, if you are happier with yourself.

Getting your needs met is up to you. And you deserve it.

3. Get Emotional Support

The need for emotional support during recovery from the Yo-Yo Syndrome is different for everyone. Some people find that they can't stick to the diet without another person's cheering them on, while others say that they'd rather keep their whole diet very private and maybe just discuss it with one or two close, supportive friends.

Whatever your particular needs, I highly recommend you attend a meeting of Overeaters Anonymous because it offers a warm, inviting means of support for Yo-Yo Syndrome sufferers. People of all types—extremely obese to the slightly overweight, young and old, men and women, educated and illiterate—find that the group offers a source of comfort and unconditional positive support.

Each group has its own unique personality, so you might have to try more than one meeting to find one you feel comfortable with. If you had tried Overeaters Anonymous in the past and decided it wasn't for you, you probably just weren't ready for it at that time, and you owe it to yourself to try the group again.

Try at least three Overeaters Anonymous meetings before you decide. The times and locations are usually listed in local newspapers, or you can call your local office of Overeaters Anonymous or Alcoholics Anonymous. If neither of these sources yield meeting information, write to the main office of Overeaters Anonymous at:

> Overeaters Anonymous
> P.O. Box 92870
> Los Angeles, CA 90009

SECTION II

This section should be worked on after you have begun the steps in Section I and have incorporated them into your lifestyle for at least two weeks. Section II is also important for your recovery from the Yo-Yo Syndrome and you should devote at least a month to the steps outlined below. And I think you'll like these steps!

1. Make Affirmations

In my practice, I give my clients a cassette tape of affirmations to listen to. Affirmations, for those unfamiliar with them, are positive statements that you can say or write over and over about yourself. You eventually incorporate these statements into your self-image and increase your self-esteem. They replace the negative self-talk you may have grown accustomed to engaging in, like "You can't do that, you'll always fail!" Such negative self-talk has equally negative effects on your daily life, because if you tell yourself you'll fail, then you're bound to do just that.

I'd like you to make your own cassette tape of affirmations using the positive statements listed below. Your own voice is the best one for the tape, because your unconscious will respond best to it. Read the statements calmly and lovingly *two times each* into a cassette (if you don't own a small portable cassette player, buy one).

Then, listen to the tape at least once a day for 30 days. At first, the statements may seem ridiculous or dishonest. That's okay—it's just a sign that your self-image is extremely negative right now. After just one week of listening to the tape daily, you'll find yourself becoming more able to accept the positive messages. At the end of a month, you'll truly believe them.

Our mind's ability to program is extremely powerful! If you don't believe this, think about the way in which you memorize songs that are played over and over. Maybe you've had this experience: you're listening to the radio and all of a sudden a song comes on that you haven't heard in 10 or 20 years. Yet you still remember all the words to the song. That's because you programmed your brain through repeated exposure to the words years ago.

Affirmations work in the same way. Here are the statements to use, remembering to state each affirmation twice into the recorder. Leave a space of approximately five seconds between each affirmation, so that you can later (when listening to the tape) repeat the affirmation to yourself:

I feel good about being who I am.

I am a lovable person, and others are attracted to me.

I achieve success in whatever I do.

I am good at sticking to something and reaching my goals.

I deserve to lose weight.

I am honest with myself and with other people, too.

I am a happy person.

I have the right to change my life to suit my personal needs.

It's okay for me to be good to myself.

I deserve happiness.

I deserve success.

I deserve to have an attractive body.

I am responsible for my own behavior.

I am responsible for what goes into my mouth.

I choose to make myself happy.

My friends are loving, successful people.

I treat myself with respect and love.

I take very good care of myself.

I enjoy exercising.

I like to have a fit body.

I pursue my goals.

Today, I'm taking steps toward a happier life.

Everyone benefits when I'm happy.

I'm responsible for how I spend the moments of my life.

I have the right to be happy and healthy.

I can put myself first without feeling guilty.

If I need something, it's okay to give it to myself.

I can ask others for help.

I enjoy losing weight.

Feeling good about myself is more important than tasting food.

I spend time in meaningful ways.

My relationship with my family has never been better.

I love myself.

Others love me, too.

I am a valuable person.

I forgive myself, and look forward to the future.

Others value me just for being who I am.

All of my dreams are coming true.

Today, I will treat myself like a queen (or king).

I deserve to be treated with respect and dignity.

I expect others to accept me.

I am open and honest.

I have fun and allow myself to relax.

I like to laugh.

I am an interesting person.

I deserve all the success life has to offer.

What matters most is what I think about myself.
I live my life according to my own beliefs and values.
I feel good about being me.
I like my body.
I deserve to lose weight.
I like being fit and trim.
It's okay for me to be admired.
It's okay for me to get compliments.
It's okay to let others get close to me.
I am a good person to get to know.
I take excellent care of myself.
I am a very special person.
I am my own best friend.
I like being with myself.
It feels good to lose weight.
The more I exercise, the more I like it.
I listen to myself and I trust myself.
I have the right to express my honest feelings.
My feelings are legitimate.
It's okay for me to feel whatever I feel.

You can also add your own affirmations to your tape. Just make sure they are worded in a positive way (e.g., I *can* stay away from overeating) as opposed to a negative way, (I *won't* overeat). If you have personal or career goals, be sure to add affirmations about them. For instance, someone who wanted to be a painter used this affirmation: "I am a successful artist," and a realtor created the affirmation, "I make $500,000 a year." Both persons made great strides in their respective careers, which they largely credit to their positive mental attitudes from listening to affirmations. These attitudes helped them to believe in their abilities to make their dreams come true. And that belief in themselves made them take steps to realize their dreams, steps that may have been too frightening for them to take had they not believed in themselves.

Make your affirmations in the present tense as if they were already true. By claiming them to be true now, you're more likely to act in such a way that will make them come true later.

2. Use Imagery

Along with reprogramming your expectations of yourself through the use of affirmations, it's also important to visually reprogram the way you see your body. I've found a definite correlation between the mental image one has of one's body and the success of any weight-loss program. Clients who never get to their goal weight very often aren't suffering from any physical weight plateau. They just can't *see themselves as a thin person!* Until you see yourself at your ideal weight, you probably won't attain it or maintain it.

This isn't anything magical or mystical; it's just that by seeing yourself as a thin person, you begin to act like a thin person. Thus, you'll choose lower-calorie meals and eat slower. You'll exercise more and take more time in grooming yourself. And in doing so, you'll create the body that you see in your mind's eye.

Many Yo-Yo Syndrome sufferers feel, deep inside, that they *can't* lose weight, as if a thin body is something out of their reach. I've heard the following over and over, "I'm so much older now than the last time I was thin—what if I'm too old to lose weight?" Although an aging body tends to have a slower metabolism, its natural state is the same as that of a young body: a normal weight. No matter what your age, you can lose weight by following the steps of this program. But first you must believe in yourself, or you'll give up before the weight has a chance to come off.

To help you edit your mental picture of your body, cut out a magazine picture of a model whose body you'd like to have. Try to find someone whose "type" (i.e., hair, eye color, height and age) is approximately the same as yours, so that you can more easily picture yourself in the model's body. Keep the picture with you and look at it often. Imagine that the model is you, and what it will feel like to have a body like his or hers. Try carrying the picture in your wallet, or tape it on your mirror or refrigerator. After a while, you may get so used to the picture that you don't even see it any longer, as if it's a piece of furniture. At that point, get a new picture to use.

You really can attain the body you desire! Many people feel they're somehow excluded from the "lucky circle" of folks who have attractive, slim bodies. They feel (I know I used to feel this way) that they're biologically barred from slimness, and that the whole idea of weight loss is absurd. Such an attitude will always prove to be self-fulfilling, so beware of your own tendency to sabotage your weight–loss program.

3. Take Inventory

Take some time to analyze your current life situation by answering the questions below. Using a notebook, spend a few hours answering these questions and writing about any feelings generated by the questions. As a Self-Esteem Eater, your weight is a symptom of underlying problems, and not the other way around. To lose weight, the underlying problems really do need to be resolved; this can't occur unless you face the problematic areas of your life and do something about them.

Analyze Your Activities. Take seven sheets of paper and label one for every day of the week. Then number each sheet 1 through 24. This represents all the hours of the day, and each day of the week. Spend the next week recording how you spent each hour of the day. For example, on the Monday sheet you may write:

12 through 7—sleeping
7 to 8—getting ready for work
8 to 9—driving to work
9 to 5—working
5 to 6—driving home from work
6 to 7—watching TV and reading newspaper
7 to 8—preparing and eating dinner

8 to 9—watching TV and getting kids ready for bed
9 to 10—reading a novel
10 to 11—getting ready for bed
11 to 12—sleeping

This exercise certainly takes time and effort to complete, but I found it extremely valuable when I first did it myself. After you are finished with your week (be sure to honestly fill in each hour), take a good look at it and ask yourself:

Am I happy with how I spent my time this week?

Were there any times I could have spent doing something different?

What thoughts kept me from spending my time differently?

What feelings kept me from spending my time differently?

Did I do anything I didn't want to this week?

Why?

If I could have three wishes that would come true, what changes would I make in my life?

What keeps me from making those changes (fear, insecurity, etc.)?

How can I begin to restructure my life so that I'm happier with it?

Is there some activity that I dream about doing, but am afraid to do?

Can I break this dream down into easier-to-realize components?

What step can I take today to make one of these components come to fruition?

Analyze Your Relationships. Next, begin to look at *whom* you spend your time with by answering these questions:

Whom do I spend most of my time with?

How would I describe this person's attitude and demeanor? (e.g., positive, negative, supportive, critical, fun, depressing, healthy, unhealthy, etc.).

How does that person's attitude affect me?

Is there someone I would like to be spending more time with?

What keeps me from being with that person?

Am I holding in feelings that need to be expressed?

Am I afraid of certain persons?

Do I have the right to choose how I spend my time?

If not, who does?

Do I give people undue power over my life, by constantly asking them for permission?

Is there someone in my life that I'd like to stay away from?

If yes, why do I punish myself by continuing to be with that person?

Do I feel I deserve to have healthy, happy relationships?

Am I more comfortable in positive or in negative relationships? (We are often most comfortable with what we're used to, even if it's negative or abusive).

Are there some changes I want to make in my relationships?

If so, what are they and what can I do today to make these changes?

Do I feel stuck in any of my relationships?

Are my feelings about this relationship affecting my eating habits and weight?

Now that you've analyzed *how* you spend your time and *whom* the time is spent with, it's time to focus on how you may want to change your activities and relationships in the future. After all, if you're not happy with how your time is spent now, how are you going to be happy in the future without making some changes in your life?

Analyze Your Goals—Part 1. Ask yourself the following questions:

What people do I admire the most?

What about them makes me admire them (e.g., fame, talent, looks, creative works, income, etc.)?

What about me is similar to these people?

What would I have to do to be more like these people?

Analyze Your Goals—Part 2. Ask yourself the following questions:

What goals (write down all of them, including weight-loss goals, things you'd like to buy, places you'd like to go, educational goals, career goals, financial goals, relationship goals, spiritual goals, etc.) would I like to have accomplished within one month?

Within six months?

Within one year?

What do I see myself doing five years from now?

What would I, ideally, like my life to be like five years from now?

Do I feel I deserve such a life?

If not, why not? (If you answered "no," then be sure to listen to your affirmations tape as often as possible to reprogram this negative belief. You definitely *do* deserve success, but first you must believe it.)

What steps can I take today toward my short-term and long-term goals?

Analyze Your Goals—Part 3. Brainstorm with yourself for just a minute and write down all of the different jobs, occupations, hobbies or avocations that you've ever admired or dreamed about (e.g., actor, lawyer, mountain climber, doctor, psychologist, writer, scuba diver, gymnast, artist, etc.). Make a list of about 25 different occupations and avocations.

Look at the list for common links among all the occupations and avocations you listed.

For instance, are they all glamorous activities that would give you lots of acknowledgment, fame or appreciation from others? If so, then this is a need of yours.

Or do all the jobs involve making big salaries and other financial rewards? If yes, then this is something that's obviously important to you.

Maybe they all involve helping others. Or they all involve working outdoors.

Whatever the common link among what you listed, it represents your own needs and values. If these needs aren't being met in your current occupation or lifestyle, then chances are you aren't satisfied.

Look again at the list. Are there one or two activities that especially appeal to you, that just seem to jump off the page because they seem so attractive? Circle those occupations or hobbies on your list (even if they seem like impossible dreams right now).

One more question: When you were a child, what did you want to be when you grew up? Why? What happened to that dream?

Seriously consider the following now that you've zeroed in on some dreams and desires: Why not enroll at the earliest opportunity in a course that will train you for your desired occupation or avocation? If you're un-sure where such courses are offered, then contact your local college and talk with a counselor there. These folks are experts at matching people with educational and training facilities, regardless of whether these people attend their institution or not. Also, public libraries usually have a section full of college catalogs. Or, ex-plore the bookstores for information about career or hobby training.

You owe it to yourself to spend the moments of your life in ways that make you happy. And for Self-Esteem Eaters, it's a *must* when it comes to achieving permanent weight loss.

5

The Stress Eaters

S TYLE NUMBER FOUR in the Yo-Yo Syndrome involves people who overeat when they
feel under the gun. I'm talking about, of course,
the Stress Eaters. Stress Eaters' weights fluctuate as a
barometer of how much pressure they're under at work
and home. When their loads are light, so are their
bodies. But when they start to feel stressed by deadlines, marital problems or a too-tight schedule, then up
go their appetites. And with the increased appetite, another upward fluctuation in weight.

That stress is created mainly by two situations that
I've seen over and over again in the lives of Stress
Eaters. The first is feeling stuck or trapped in some area
of life. The second is having an overdone lifestyle.

The Stress Eater must resolve his or her troublesome situation rather than attempt to ease the stress with food. Overeating, of course, only *adds* to your stress level, because it makes you feel angry at yourself, fat, unattractive and lethargic. This chapter will help you discover other alternatives to relieve stress.

Feeling Stuck, Feeling Fat

There are as many areas that people feel stuck in as there are people, but in general Yo-Yo Syndrome sufferers tend to get stuck in these ruts more than in others: marriages and occupations.

FEELING STUCK IN MARRIAGES

Jenny had been married to George, her second husband, for 12 years. "I knew before I married him that things between George and me weren't all that great," the 36-year-old nurse told me. "But I just keep hanging on, thinking things would change or get better soon."

When Jenny related her unhappiness with her husband and described how he belittled and insulted her, she also explained that she was afraid to lose George's financial support if she were to divorce him. She was terrified she'd lose the house and be unable to support their three young children. Though she worked and had her own moderate source of income, Jenny chose to stay in a psychologically abusive marriage rather than risk a financially impoverished lifestyle.

Many women find themselves in Jenny's shoes, and feel helpless to do anything to change the situation—and turn to the refrigerator or kitchen cupboard to temporarily mask their pain.

Women, of course, aren't the only ones who feel stuck in empty marriages. Men have their fair share as well. Many share a story similar to Ray's: A 40-year-old engineer, Ray had married his high school sweetheart, Gloria, right after graduating from college. Ray was extremely devoted to Gloria, and he put a lot of energy into trying to keep her happy—no easy task, as Ray found out during the course of his marriage.

"I don't know what I'm doing wrong," Ray complained, "and I don't know what else I could possibly do to make her happy!" He described spending hundreds of dollars a month on Gloria's wardrobe and on dining out several times a week. "I really do everything I can think of, and I buy Gloria whatever she wants. But no matter what I do, she's never satisfied. All she does is complain about what a lousy husband I am, and demand that I make more money to satisfy her needs."

Ray found that the more frustrated he became with Gloria's insatiable appetite for clothes and other expensive endeavors, the more he'd turn to food to soothe his feelings of being an inadequate husband. Ray didn't want to divorce Gloria, but he wasn't happy with their relationship either. Feeling helpless to make the situation any better—"It's really been this way for 20 years, why should it change now?"—Ray felt stuck with no way out, a feeling that was putting ten pounds a year on his already overweight frame.

Often not trusting their own ability to make the right decision about their marriages, Stress Eaters stay for years hoping that things will change for the better somehow. And they turn to food to deal with the powerful feelings experienced in such unsatisfying marriages. One client, married for the third time, told me that during each of her marriages she had gained over 30 pounds. "I realize that I ate during those marriages, as well as in this marriage, because I feel dead inside. Somehow, the food makes it all not seem so bad for a while."

FEELING STUCK IN OCCUPATIONS

Donna was a lawyer who wished she'd never heard of the occupation. Hating paperwork, debates and the pressure of deadlines, Donna was as mismatched as anyone could be for her line of work. In fact, the only thing that kept Donna in her profession was the huge salary it commanded from the law firm she worked for.

"I'm trapped, absolutely trapped," Donna explained. "Between the mortgage payments on my house, college tuition for my two kids, and putting food on the table, I need every dime I make. So how can I quit and start over in another profession?" Every morning, Donna would wake up with dread in her heart—dread about having to go to the office or to court one more time.

She'd drag herself to work after eating a large breakfast, then she'd eat continuously all day long. "It's the only way I can handle the pressure," Donna told me.

Jill had every confidence in her abilities to run the health club she owned and make a lot of money in the process. The problem was, owning a successful gym wasn't making Jill happy in the way she'd always dreamed it would. "It's kind of an empty feeling," Jill told me, "considering all those years I'd worked so hard to put this thing together. Now that I've realized my goal, I think, 'Big deal'." The anti-climactic emptiness she was experiencing is normal in successful individuals who feel as if they've climbed the mountain, and wonder "What next?"

I've seen so many clients who felt stuck in their careers because an exaggerated need for job security made them ignore the fact that they hated the work they were doing. Al, for example, really wanted to return to tending bar—a job he'd held in college—but was afraid of disappointing his father. "Dad always tells me my government job is the most secure position in the world. He says he's really proud of me for getting this nice, secure job."

Another client, Kim, worked for an aerospace firm in the insurance department. "I really don't like the work I do," she told me. "It's boring and my boss is a real jerk."

"Why don't you look around for another job?" I asked.

"Well, only 8 more years and I'll retire," was Kim's explanation.

FEELING STUCK IN OTHER AREAS

While most people feel stuck in their jobs or marriages, there are other areas Stress Eaters often feel trapped in.

For instance, 33-year-old Nicole didn't know how to escape the way her mother tried to control her life. Nicole's mother called at least once a day and lectured her daughter on eating, working, talking to people, and every other imaginable subject. "I'd love to tell her off," Nicole said, "but I'm afraid what it would do to her health."

Eating to cover up a problem does not improve any situation, as most of us know; it merely gives us short-term relief when a long-term plan to rectify the situation is really what's called for. Are you stuck? If so, some of the questions below may help crystallize your thinking about the problem enough to help you form a plan of action—followed, of course, by the footwork necessary to carry the plan to fruition.

In what areas of your life do you feel stuck?

What is negative about the situation that makes you want to change it?

What is positive about the situation that makes you want to stay where you are?

What scares you about changing your situation?

Are there steps you can take to improve your situation so you won't want to leave? (This doesn't include hoping or wishing things will get better.)

Are there steps you can take today to help you change or leave your situation?

Are you, at all, waiting for someone to give you permission to take these steps? If so, who? Why do you feel you need someone else's approval to change or improve your own life?

How does feeling stuck affect your eating?

The Overdone Lifestyle

If your schedule is crammed full of too many things to do, and you never have enough time to get everything done, you may be experiencing the second major cause of stress, an overdone lifestyle. Stress arises as you rush from task to task, trying to beat the clock to get everything accomplished. If you suffer from an overdone lifestyle, you don't take enough time to care properly for yourself, you probably don't get enough rest or exercise, and your eating likely consists of haphazard meals at fast-food restaurants. In addition, you probably reel from the momentum and don't know how to slow down your frantic pace. This makes you especially vulnerable to overeating, because you may use meals and snacks as an excuse to stop working for a while.

My client Jennifer had an overdone lifestyle. The 33-year-old business owner spent most of each therapy session complaining about all the things she was expected to do at home and work. The book work and inventory control. The taxes and payroll. Making sure her children got up on time each morning, and then dressing and feeding them breakfast before the school

bus arrived. After work, she'd try to find time to play
with her kids and help them with homework. Somewhere in between all this, Jennifer would fix dinner and
she and her husband, an attorney, would clean the
house and get the kids bathed and into bed.

After that, Jennifer would try to unwind by beginning an evening "snack" that normally lasted until
"The Tonight Show" went off the air. When Jennifer
first saw me about losing weight, she believed that she
was a victim of a schedule that left her no choice but to
run herself ragged and then overeat late at night.

However, in examining the tasks she had to do, Jennifer saw clearly that she was performing them out of
choice. *She* was the master-planner of her hectic days
and evenings. Although she could readily afford to get
help for herself—a bookkeeper for her business and a
house cleaning service for her home—she hadn't given
herself permission to do so. This realization was uncomfortable for Jennifer to face, because it implied she
was responsible for creating and organizing how her
time was spent; no outside entity was forcing her to do
this or that.

Did Jennifer, after realizing her involvement in her
overdone lifestyle, decide to live a simpler life? No. At
least, not right away. Jennifer first looked at why she
needed to stay busy and productive: She was afraid not
to be. Working, regardless of whether that meant balancing her checkbook, sweeping the floor or managing
the horticulture business she ran from her home, was
how Jennifer defined herself. If she wasn't working, she

felt somehow worthless. And guilty. As if she were bad.

Jennifer feared that if she slowed her pace at all, something horrible might happen. This vague fear involved worry that she'd be judged by others as lazy—a fear stemming from being raised by workaholic parents who pushed her to keep busy.

"The only time I got their attention was when I brought home straight A's on my report card," Jennifer recalled with a tense expression on her face. "I remember this one time, I had all A's, except for a B in math. My Dad took one look at that B and told me I should try harder next time. He didn't even say anything about all the A's I had gotten in the other classes!"

With such high stakes—her parents' attention, approval and what felt like their love—riding on Jennifer's academic performance, the young girl began to feel as if she was loved *for what she did, and not for who she was.* She, like her parents, began to give herself conditional love. If she didn't do things perfectly, Jennifer would chastise herself. If she did things well, Jennifer would momentarily congratulate herself and then go right on to another project. By the time I met her at age 33, Jennifer's daily schedule was an endless list of back-to-back projects, errands and appointments. And even though she was a very accomplished young woman who owned her own business, Jennifer felt as if it wasn't enough.

Enough for what? For the approval she craved from her father and mother. A reassurance from her father that he was proud of her. A hug from Mom to let

Jennifer know she was appreciated as a person. And, most of all, the knowledge that both parents loved her, and that she was a lovable person.

The Yo-Yo Syndrome Diet for Jennifer was difficult because it meant coming to terms with the knowledge that her parents weren't capable of giving her the love and approval she sought. Jennifer realized that this didn't mean she was unworthy or unlovable (something she feared). It *did* mean, however, that Jennifer would have to provide her own love and approval instead of relying on her parents.

Was Jennifer then able to let go of her overdone lifestyle? Well . . . no, not yet. She was still too scared to relinquish her hectic schedule although she would tell me she *wished* she could let herself relax. Jennifer wasn't yet totally convinced that she'd profit from a more relaxed lifestyle.

The phone call came on a Monday morning. "Doreen," she told me, "something's wrong! I need to see you right away." We scheduled an emergency session for an hour later, and what I heard from Jennifer was not surprising. She, like other Stress Eaters with overdone lifestyles, was finding that she was pushing herself much too hard and her body was beginning to protest.

That morning, she'd had a panic attack. Common among people who drive themselves past exhaustion, a panic attack involves a racing heart, waves of dizziness, light-headedness, an inability to catch one's breath—as if the lungs had holes in them—and a fear that one is dying, having a heart attack or going crazy. When I explained what had happened to Jennifer, she seemed relieved but worried that it might happen again. "What do I do now?" she asked. Jennifer had finally hit bottom and was ready to learn how to relax.

After going to a physician for a checkup, Jennifer took a week off from work. During that week, I asked Jennifer to compose a brutally honest list of her priorities. Once she'd done that, we looked at which activities Jennifer could cut out of her schedule. All activities that diverted her from her priorities were cut. Times for play and relaxation were scheduled in. Once Jennifer accepted that her health depended on a balanced, sane lifestyle ("After all, I won't get as much done if I die early," she told me), she let herself slow down.

Today, Jennifer is a different woman from the one I first met. She looks wonderful after losing the 30 extra pounds she carried from continual snacking, and her face has lost the tense lines and stern look it used to carry. But most of all, Jennifer is happy with herself today and no longer loves herself conditionally.

If the beginning of Jennifer's story sounds at all like your own, rest assured you're not alone. Having an overdone lifestyle is a big part of being a Stress Eater, but it's also extremely difficult to give up. It feels frightening, as if you might lose some ground you've gained. Slowing down can seem tantamount to admitting you're weak and can't stand the pressure. As if you've failed before you've had a chance to prove yourself.

As mentioned before, though, slowing down doesn't mean letting go of productivity or worthwhile activities. Actually, it means increasing both while at the

same time letting go of the hundreds of meaningless
tasks that eat up your day and end up frustrating you.
You know—those activities that leave you feeling resentful and empty after you perform them. The ones
that make you want to eat.

Step #1 for Stress Eaters:
Evaluate and Reduce Stress

The best way to reschedule your day to allow for a
more relaxed lifestyle *yet still get the important things accomplished* is to make a list of priorities. I highly recommend you do this. On a sheet of paper, write down
the five or ten things that you value most in life. These
could be goals ("Finish that M.B.A. degree by next
year"), objectives ("Pay off the charge cards"), desires
("Feel better about myself"), values ("Spend more time
playing with the children") or concerns ("Take better
care of my health").

What is on your list is not as important as the honesty
of your list. Many people are ashamed to admit, for
example, that their family, health or religious beliefs are
not at the top of their list. But if they aren't, they aren't,
and that's how the list should be written. If it's a list
written according to what you think "should" be on it,
the list will be worthless because it won't be *your* list.
Remember, also, that you don't need to show this list
to anyone else.

After you write down your priorities, write down

the approximate number of hours you spend every week pursuing each priority. For example, if you put "Finishing my degree" as your number one priority, write down how many hours you spend in school and spend studying each week. Then write the hours spent on the other priorities on your list.

After you finish, you may be surprised—or horrified —to find that you don't spend many hours on the things that are important to you. No wonder you feel frustrated, as if you're spinning your wheels and not getting anywhere!

Your schedule, ideally, will show that the largest part of your time is spent on your first priority, followed by your second priority and so forth. What's that you say? "Impossible?" Well, I've heard that before—and I've found it's usually much more possible than people realize. It's just that they're not used to giving themselves permission to have a life full of activities that make them happy. Unfortunately, many people are like Jennifer; they have to hit bottom with their health before they decide to change their lives. But you don't need to.

The following exercises may at first glance seem morbid or depressing, but they are designed to help you continue examining your priorities. My clients who've tried both exercises report they're tremendously helpful in clarifying what's really important to them; in addition, these exercises motivate them to readjust their lives in order to live according to their priorities.

Exercise 1

Imagine the phone rings and you answer. It's your doctor with some distressing news: the results of your last physical exam are in and your prognosis is grim. You have just three more months to live. During these last months of your life, you'll retain all your present physical capabilities and you won't feel any signs of ill health. But at the end of three months, it'll all be over.

Stunned, you hang up the phone. What changes will you make in your life *right now* to make your last three months more enjoyable? What's the first answer that pops into your head?

Of course no one knows how much time each of us has left on earth; it could be an hour or decades. Yet, most of us live as if we've got an eternity left. We procrastinate changing our lives, as if tomorrow—when that perfect moment comes—we'll get started on what we want to do. We act like children waiting for our parents to give us permission to live our own lives. And as a result we end up putting up with unnecessary frustration.

We often don't see that it's up to us to change things we don't like, because it's scary to take responsibility for our own lives. Now ask yourself these questions:

What changes did I think about during this exercise?
How did I feel when thinking about taking the risk and making those changes?
What keeps me from making those changes now?

How is my eating affected by my feelings about my present lifestyle?

Exercise 2

Write your own obituary or notice of death as you'd like it to appear in the newspaper upon your demise. Include in it all the accomplishments you'd someday like to achieve, but of course in the past tense:

Jane Smith will be remembered as an entrepreneur who rose above incredible odds to build an empire of grocery store chains and restaurants across America. She spent her last years helping various charities build homes for the homeless through many large donations. She also erected the "Jane Smith Library" in this town for use by handicapped children.

While it may sound like a morbid project, writing your own obituary is extremely helpful in clarifying just what it is you want to get done in your short lifespan. Of course, no one enjoys thinking about his or her own mortality, but by being realistic in assessing approximately how much time you've got left in this life and figuring how long it will take you to achieve your goals, you can plan how wise or unwise it is to put off working toward them.

Many people fear being labeled selfish by spending money or time on self-improvement or leisure. Taking time from your family and friends and spending money to further your goals isn't selfish; it's merely a way for you to improve your life and the lives of those around you.

As a matter of fact, when Yo-Yo Syndrome sufferers aren't happy with their lives, when they're living to please others and not themselves, they are particularly difficult to live with. The resentment and depression that spring from not liking yourself or your life rub off on your children, your spouse and other people.

On the other hand, if you're happy and satisfied with your life, you'll be a pleasure to be around. You'll also be an inspiration to your children, teaching them values about life that will help them have happy adulthoods, too.

Now, is that being selfish?

It is important to understand what to do when you feel stuck or live an overdone lifestyle because both are intimately connected with overeating. You don't need to radically or impulsively change your life or slow your pace entirely. What you must do, however, is examine how you feel about your life and the way you spend your time. Be very honest with yourself during this assessment, and if you are truly dissatisfied, take one or two small steps to make your situation better.

It's also important to become acutely aware of how your eating ties in with your stress level. For Stress Eaters, like Emotion Eaters, the best way to gain awareness is through a journal. Make the time to keep a personal diary of how you feel before, during and after you eat. After keeping the journal for two weeks, look for patterns in your overeating by asking yourself:

Do I eat more during the work week or on weekends?

Is this tied in to feeling more stressed at home, or at work?

Are there certain times of the day when I overeat?

If yes, is this because I'm using food as a stress-management tool?

Do I use food to procrastinate, because I feel I've got too many things to do?

A More Relaxed and Thinner Lifestyle

Stress is a symptom of a pressured lifestyle, one that involves worry mixed with both monotony and risk-taking. When you're stressed, you're living on the edge of your seat, taking a toll on your body—and on your eating.

Many people enjoy a hurried lifestyle—to them, it's not stressful to be juggling four projects at once. Instead, they find it stimulating and exciting. So stress is a subjective and personal state of being, and everyone's definition of it is different.

As mentioned before, I've found that many Stress Eaters are reluctant to give up their stress-filled lifestyles. For instance, 27-year-old Lynn had her sights set on an upper management position at the firm where she worked. To try to get the promotion, Lynn worked overtime every day, volunteered to be on various company committees, and knocked herself out trying to be visible to her superiors. In general, Lynn's life revolved around obtaining her goal.

When Lynn came to me for help with her Yo-Yo Syndrome, it was clear to me her overdone lifestyle played a big part in her overeating habits. Every night, she'd unwind with a two-hour-long "snack," which Lynn justified by complaining that she was too keyed-up after work to cook a normal dinner for herself. These snacks, as far as I could estimate, were adding an extra 1000 to 1500 calories to her daily total. So it was no wonder that Lynn constantly struggled with an extra 30 pounds.

When I suggested that we look for ways to loosen up her pressure-cooker lifestyle, however, Lynn immediately became defensive. "If I don't work this hard," she shot back, "I'll never make it to the vice presidency!" To Lynn, stress and success seemed one and the same; you could not get one without the other.

Other Stress Eaters feel their stress-filled lives aren't optional. One of my clients, 33-year-old Buffy, told me she felt guilty when she's not doing something around the house. Buffy said she didn't realize she could *choose* whether or not to have a stressful life—to her it seemed an externally mandated lifestyle. In addition, she felt that she'd need "permission" from some authority before she could relax. And ambitious Lynn, described above, was afraid she'd miss out on success if she relaxed at all.

Many people, fortunately, are discovering it is possible to have a relaxing lifestyle and still derive the emotional and material pleasures they value from life. I've found that most Stress Eaters can add two dimensions to their lives and find an immediate reduction in their stress levels. The first is increasing the amount of fun in their lives. The second is spending more time out-of-doors.

This book isn't really broad enough to provide a lot of information on stress reduction; there are many excellent books on the subject available. In addition, professional counselors can help you restructure your life to reduce stress.

But if you are a Stress Eater, you can easily take some of the pressure off of you by adopting the two suggestions—have fun and get outside more often—and implementing them at least once a week. Spending time outdoors has a soothing effect on overtired executives and office workers who spend so much time indoors and in cars.

Having fun helps also, because it allows Stress Eaters to break loose from the rigid structure that 9-to-5 worklives are made of. Why not go to the park and swing on the swings? Or chase someone around the room and then tickle them? When was the last time you flew a kite? Went to an amusement park or a comedy movie? Or laughed really hard? What can you do today to add some fun to your life?

Stress is a fact of life from time to time for all of us. And, of course, not all stress is bad—it can be tremendously motivating. But one thing is true about stress for all Yo-Yo Syndrome sufferers: If you feel pressured, rushed or stressed, you shouldn't eat over it. As you read along, you'll discover alternatives to using food as an answer to your stress. You can also make your own list of food-alternatives to keep handy (perhaps on the refrigerator door) when you want to eat because of stress. The list could spell out all those projects you've been wanting to get to but never have time for, such as this list:

MY FOOD-ALTERNATIVE LIST

1. Write letter to Aunt Mary.
2. Clean out closet.
3. Call around to compare insurance rates.
4. Go shopping for bookshelf.
5. Make appointment for haircut.
6. Start making the lace pillow for Sis.

It's a good idea to include one or two pleasant activities on the food-alternative list, too. Use this list to divert your attention when your hunger pangs originate from your stress and not from your stomach. In this way, you'll feel good about spending your time in pleasant, meaningful ways while you avoid overeating.

Other Choices to Make

Stress Eaters, in order to lose weight, are basically left with two choices: They can de-stress their lives to reduce their overeating, or they can keep their lifestyles as they are, and turn to a healthier way to control their stress level.

The section above dealt with the first choice, but some Stress Eaters may not be ready to let go of areas in their lives that produce stress. For these folks, it's vital they turn to something other than food to alleviate the turmoil and pressure triggered by a stuck or over-done lifestyle.

There are degrees of both positive and negative ways to deal with stress (other than eliminating the source of stress), as demonstrated by this continuum:

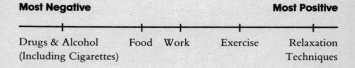

WAYS TO DEAL WITH STRESS

Most Negative   **Most Positive**

Drugs & Alcohol   Food   Work   Exercise   Relaxation
(Including Cigarettes)   Techniques

Drugs, alcohol, food and work (many people throw themselves into their work in response to stress) are ineffective ways to combat stress, as most people are aware. Most of the time, these things make the situation worse instead of better. People turn to them, of course, because they provide immediate short-term relief of stress and psychological pain. However, after the effect wears off, the stress returns.

Exercise, in contrast, is an extremely positive method for stress control. It not only helps to "cathart" or get

rid of pent-up anger and resentment, but it also helps to
build up resistance to future stress. People who exercise
regularly find that they are less irritated by the little
irksome things in life than they were before they
adopted an exercise program. Chapter 9 outlines other
aspects of exercise, but for now, Stress Eaters should
plan on incorporating some sort of fitness routine into
their schedule as a way to manage stress and keep the
weight off.

If you're a Stress Eater, one of the best things you can
do for yourself to reduce your stress level *and* reduce
your Stress Eating is to begin an exercise program. This
means exercising regularly four or five times a week,
for at least 40 minutes each time. The exercise can be
anything—jogging, walking, swimming, tennis or
aerobics—but it must get your heart rate elevated and
work your major muscle groups in order to effectively
help you lose weight and reduce your stress level.

Many Stress Eaters find that stopping off at the gym
on the way to or from work is the best way to fit
exercise into their crammed schedules. Corinne, for instance, had tried going to the gym many times in the
past but had always quit because it seemed so time-
consuming. "I'd get home from work and the last thing
I'd want to do was to change into my leotard and drive
back across town to the gym," she remembered.
"Now," she says, "I keep my gym clothes and tennis
shoes in my car and go right after work. That way, I
don't have any excuse to avoid exercising."

Since most Stress Eaters turn to food at the end of
their workday, exercising after work is an excellent way

of avoiding the urge to eat. Corinne told me she's inspired to stay on her Yo-Yo Syndrome Diet when she goes to the gym and sees all the women with beautiful figures working out around her. "I want to look as good as they do," Corinne says, "and I know I can if I exercise and stay away from snacking at night."

Melissa, another one of my clients who goes to the gym after work, tells me exercising helps her work off the upsetting feelings that build up in her stressful job as a customer service representative for a department store. "It's great!" she exclaimed. "While I'm riding on the stationary bike, I'll be thinking about all the customers who upset me during the day. With each pump on the bicycle, I can feel the anger draining out of my body."

Where before Melissa would take her anger and stress out on food in her refrigerator, she now finds that exercising puts things into perspective for her. "By the time I leave the gym, whatever was bugging me seems small and insignificant," Melissa says.

If you don't have an exercise program, take steps to begin one. Many people argue they don't have time to go to a gym. In truth, those who exercise find they actually have more time because of the increased energy they feel from all the physical activity. They also have more time in their day because they spend less time eating and worrying. And after a month of regular workouts, most find they love exercising. Chapter 9 delves further into the subject of beginning a fitness routine.

The Art of Relaxing

Relaxation techniques, once considered something for those who practiced "alternative lifestyles," are now a proven method for reducing stress levels and increasing physical health, especially in the face of stress. In fact, a recent study of longevity concluded that using relaxation techniques twice a week was as effective as quitting smoking in increasing life expectancy. Relaxation techniques were even more effective than exercise!

The two methods together—exercise plus regular deep relaxation—are ideal for Stress Eaters. Both will help you develop new habits for dealing with stress, habits that in the long run will end up reducing your stress level.

Probably the easiest way to begin a relaxation program is to purchase a cassette tape labeled with a title such as "Relaxation" or "Self-Hypnosis." These are usually located in the educational or special-interest section of the cassette tape displays in major bookstores. Buy a tape with an audible—as opposed to subliminal—voice track on it. While the music or sounds on subliminal tapes tend to be relaxing, the whole idea of subliminal learning has been discredited. Studies show that voices and pictures must be consciously audible and visible before the information can go into the brain. Any benefits you receive from subliminal materials, although real, are because of the placebo effect, or power of suggestion.

In contrast, audible tapes can teach you how to relax yourself by learning the methods of step-by-step deep muscle relaxation and guided imagery. Basically, these tapes will help you to: slowly relax each muscle in your body, one by one; relax your mind and let go of worries; and create a relaxing image in your mind, such as sitting on the beach watching a sunset.

Once you purchase the tape, it's important to actually use it. Many Stress Eaters buy a relaxation tape and then put it on the shelf after only a few uses. You'll need to schedule in your relaxation just as you do everything else in your life.

Take the time to relax . . . you've worked hard and you deserve a break! And most importantly, the next time you feel hungry, wait 15 minutes to see if it isn't stress that's making you want to eat. If it is stress, remember that food is not an option for you to use in managing your stress. Exercise is an option. Listening to your relaxation tape is an option. But eating is not.

In the next chapter, we'll look at Style Number Five in the Yo-Yo Syndrome: The Snowball Effect Eaters, who find their portions growing larger and larger until they regain all their weight one more time.

6

The Snowball Effect Eaters

IF YOU picture a snowball gathering momentum, speed and size as it rolls down the side of a snowy mountain, you'll begin to get a feel for Style Number Five in the Yo-Yo Syndrome. This is the dieter who yo-yos because of food portions that grow in size, like the rolling snowball.

Phyllis had been gaining and losing 15 to 25 pounds since she'd entered college ten years ago. The 28-year-old elementary school teacher had first put on weight as a college freshman, mostly because she overate to deal with the pressures of term papers and final exams and the frightening feeling of being 500 miles away from home.

Her first diet was given to her by the college nurse.

"It was one of those hospital-based diet sheets," Phyllis remembered. "I followed it to the letter and and ate exactly what the diet sheet told me to, which wasn't exactly easy considering I was eating all my meals at a college cafeteria." Phyllis easily shed the 20 pounds she'd gained, and after she was able to fit back into her old jeans she quickly abandoned the diet.

The weight came back on in one semester and Phyllis was horrified when she found, for the second time in her life, that she couldn't fit into her clothes. "So, I went back to the college nurse and asked for another diet sheet," she explained. "But this time, the nurse recommended that I join a diet club since I hadn't been able to keep the weight off." And so she did.

The diet club, which met on campus, helped Phyllis commit herself to losing weight again. "The support was great," she recalled. "It was nice seeing I wasn't the only one who was struggling to keep my grades up and my weight down." The club's recommended eating plan seemed easy for Phyllis to follow after her previous experience with the stringent and bland hospital-based diet. This time, the weight took a little longer to come off, but Phyllis did lose the 20 pounds.

What happened after that was typical of Snowball Effect Eaters. "I was determined not to put the weight back on again, so I continued to follow the diet club's eating plan," Phyllis explained. She stopped going to the meetings and assumed that as long as she followed the same menus, her weight would no longer present a problem. Imagine her shock when, six months later,

Phyllis found she'd not only regained the 20 pounds but an additional 5 pounds on top of that!

By the time I met Phyllis, she'd been yo-yoing like this for ten years. Together, Phyllis and I examined her history of weight losses and gains, and looked at each experience in detail until a clear pattern emerged. Phyllis would lose weight following diet programs that spelled out specific 900- to 1200-calorie menus. She'd get in the habit of eating the breakfasts, lunches and dinners in each diet until she'd lose her excess weight. At that point, Phyllis would continue following the diet but with one important difference: she'd become a "sloppy-portion eater." That is, she'd become inattentive in her portion control.

For example, if the diet told her to eat three ounces of lean beef, a plain baked potato and a green salad with diet dressing, Phyllis would follow the diet exactly while shedding the excess weight. As soon as she'd reached her goal weight, though, the meal would look more like this: six ounces of steak, one-half baked potato with sour cream, and a green salad with thousand island dressing. Within a few months the "same" dinner would consist of a huge slab of marbled steak, a whole baked potato with butter and sour cream, and a heaping bowl of salad laden with cheese, pasta, croutons and blue cheese dressing. Phyllis would increase her portions gradually and wouldn't notice how much she was deviating from the "core" meal her diets had propounded. That is, she wouldn't notice until she had regained her excess weight.

We know from some well-constructed studies done

on Yo-Yo Syndrome sufferers that continual fluctuations in weight from on-again, off-again dieting plays havoc on a person's body and metabolism. The evidence is clear that every time a person diets, weight loss becomes subsequently slower. Perhaps the first time you dieted you noticed that you reached your goal weight rather rapidly. The next time, maybe you noted that the weight loss was somewhat slower. And the diet following that one may have seemed to take an eternity to produce results.

After years and years of dieting, our bodies learn—almost like in the story of "The Boy Who Cried Wolf"—that the food deprivation during the diet is only going to be temporary. The body of a long-term Yo-Yo Syndrome sufferer, almost from the moment that the new diet is started, goes into a state of "holding on to" each calorie it is fed. The metabolism slows way down, and weight loss seems to take forever. This is a most frustrating situation for Snowball Effect Eaters, who find themselves in a perplexingly perpetual state of gaining and losing weight.

Snowball Effect Varieties

Snowball Effect Eaters often gain weight because they mistakenly believe that once they are thin, they can eat whatever they want. My 35-year-old client Pam, for example, had attained her goal weight after four months of following a diet she'd found in a woman's magazine.

She assumed that the role of the diet was to help her *lose* weight. "Now that I'm thin," Pam reasoned, "I can eat like a normal person again."

The only problem was that Pam based her idea of a normal person's eating habits on an abnormal conception. Pam's slender husband, Gary, and equally slim 14-year-old son, Tim, could eat whatever they wanted and not gain any weight. "I figured I'd eat whatever Gary and Tim ate," Pam explained. "I mean *they* never gained any weight, so I thought if I ate exactly the same as them, I'd be as thin as they were."

So Pam ate as many fried pork chops, french fries and pieces of dessert as her husband and son. If Gary ate a one-pound steak, so would Pam. If Tim had a stack of pancakes for breakfast, Pam would follow suit. Of course, it didn't take long for Pam to realize that her metabolism was much different from the rest of her family's—after she ended up regaining the 30 pounds she'd so diligently dieted away. I call Snowball Effect Eaters like Pam "backpedalers" because they remind me of cyclists who work so hard to ride their bicycles up a hill, only to abandon their efforts and goals by not pedalling any more. Backpedalers, such as Pam, slide right back into overeating.

Another Snowball Effect Eater, Jackie, a 42-year-old homemaker, had the same experience every time she dieted: she rapidly grew bored of what seemed to be one montonous diet after another. "I can only take so much broiled fish before I start to scream!" Jackie said. The longest period Jackie had ever been able to stick to a diet was two months. After that, she'd go off the diet to eat what she called "real food."

Jackie was a "recreational eater," that is, she viewed eating in the same way that many see hobbies or vacations—it was her way of having fun. "I just *love* to eat!" she exclaimed. "There's nothing better on earth than a delicious meal."

Jackie's Yo-Yo Syndrome Diet Plan necessitated her adding alternative, as well as healthier, forms of entertainment. Reluctantly at first, she joined a tennis class as a way to have fun, exercise and meet new friends. With the thrill of several successes in that venture, Jackie had the courage to sign up for a course in stained glass and another one in photography.

These new activities created fun in Jackie's life, filled in her previously uneventful days with structure, and provided her with new friends and interesting things to do. As a result, Jackie found it much easier to stick to her Yo-Yo Syndrome Diet.

Another type of Snowball Effect Eater is the "seasonal eater." This is the person who gains weight only during certain seasons of the year, usually winter. Roxanne had no trouble shedding pounds during the spring, and she kept her figure looking great right up until the first autumn leaf fell. But right around October of each year, Roxanne's appetite would go out of control.

Seasonal eaters, like Roxanne, fall prey to this phenomenon for various reasons. Some find that the cold winter months mean less physical activity and more time sitting indoors, thus leading to more opportunity to eat and fewer ways to burn off the calories. Others succumb to the pressures to eat that go hand-in-hand with Halloween, Thanksgiving, Christmas and New Year's. After all, at what other time of year do you have four holidays that are centered on eating so close together? And centered on eating fattening foods, at that? Still other seasonal eaters feel they lose motivation for dieting during the winter. For them, as soon as bathing suit season is over, all reasons for wanting to be thin vanish as they cloak their heavier bodies in sweaters and wool skirts or pants.

Still another variety in Style Number Five of the Yo-Yo Syndrome is the "sneak eater." These people play a game with themselves while dieting, a kind of "sleight of hands." The scenario of the sneak eater is often like that of Irma, who was constantly beginning, ending, or on a diet.

Irma would always begin her diets with the best of intentions. "This time," she'd promise herself, "I'll be good and follow the diet exactly." She'd diet down to within ten pounds of her goal weight, and then something would almost snap inside of her. The 33-year-old receptionist would eat something off her diet. A banana split or a package of doughnuts. Anything, as long as it wasn't allowed on her diet. And always, Irma would feel deliciously wicked, as if she was being a naughty girl.

The next day, Irma would anxiously step on her bathroom scale to assess the damages from her feast. And lo and behold, her weight would still be the same! Irma would glow with a warm satisfaction that she'd gotten away with her diet cheating. This led her to plan other cheats, that unfortunately, got closer and closer together. Eventually, of course, her continuous over-eating of high-calorie desserts caught up with Irma and she regained the weight. Irma hadn't gotten away with anything but another cycle of feeling frustrated and fat.

One other variety of the Snowball Effect Eater is the "attention-shy eater"—someone who, when she loses weight, becomes afraid of being a thin person and eats more to escape back into the safety of her fat body. Betty was such a person. When I first met her, she complained that her dieting never took her below 150 pounds. No matter what she did, every time she got to 150 pounds, she'd go off her diet and start overeating again.

Upon examination of Betty's pattern of weight losses and gains, we found her plateaus weren't physical in origin—they were psychological. It turned out that at around 150 pounds, Betty's male co-workers would begin to pay sexual attention to her. They'd whistle and admire her. They'd whoop catcalls when she'd walk by. And one man even asked her out for a date. Betty, who was already struggling to keep her marriage intact, was afraid of her own reactions to all the male attention she got when she slimmed down. She felt flattered, but at the same time frightened (some of it was fear that she'd lose control and have an affair with her suitor). Betty's weight gains occurred because, unconsciously, she felt more at ease when she was overweight.

Then, too, there is the "apathy eater," who loses motivation while dieting. This was a real problem for Crystal, an attractive 35-year-old brunette cosmetolo-

gist who had yo-yoed since she'd been a teenager. "The
problem," Crystal explained to me, "is that half the
time I just stop caring whether I'm fat or not. I always
start my diet because I can't fit into my clothes anymore, and I always tell myself that 'this time it will be
different; this time I'll lose the whole thirty extra
pounds.'

"But it never fails!" Crystal shook her head and
sighed deeply. "I'll get ten or twelve pounds off and
then I'll give up trying after that. I wish I could stay
motivated to get those other twenty pounds off for
once."

Step #1 for Snowball Effect Eaters: Get the Mindset

All Snowball Effect Eaters need one major ingredient in
their lives to stop the up-and-down weight fluctuations
of their Yo-Yo Syndromes: continuous motivation to
lose weight and then keep the weight off. Permanent
weight loss is a long-term goal, but it's difficult to keep
the rewards of such an endeavor in mind when facing
the immediate gratification from eating. The 28 tips
below are designed to help Snowball Effect Eaters
maintain the needed commitment, if not enthusiasm,
necessary in the Yo-Yo Syndrome Diet.

1. Ask yourself: *Why* am I trying to lose weight?
Do I want to lose weight to please someone else

(lover, spouse, parent, etc.)? Or do I want to slim down to please myself?

These are extremely important questions, because the answers have a lot to do with how your diet will go. Unless you are trying to lose weight to please yourself, it's going to be tough to keep your motivation level high. Do it for yourself, not someone else! After all, what's important is whether or not *you* are happy with yourself.

2. Get in the habit of weighing yourself every morning, right after you wake up and after you've urinated. Don't skip a single day, because by weighing yourself daily you'll get immediate feedback about how your eating plan (described in the next chapter) is affecting your weight. If you don't weigh yourself daily, you might slip into denial about the weight you're gaining. Or you might become complacent about your progressively larger meals. The reality of the numbers on the scale, then, helps to focus your attention on your need to diet.

3. Write your goal weight (i.e., 115 pounds, 135 pounds, etc.) in bright ink on a large piece of paper, and hang it where you'll see it when you weigh yourself in the morning. That way, any discrepancy between the two numbers—the one on the scale and the one on the paper—will help keep you motivated to lose weight.

4. Stop thinking that diets have a beginning and an ending. Instead, when you begin the eating plan described in the next chapter, think of a total and permanent change in lifestyle and eating habits. A healthy, attractive body isn't something you achieve and then stop working on. Rather, dieting is a process and a journey instead of a goal to attain.

5. Related to this is the importance of positive thinking while you're dieting. Instead of thinking that you're depriving yourself when you say "no" to fattening food, turn it into a positive thought by remembering that you're really saying "yes" to a slim, healthy body. And "yes" to feeling proud about how you look.

6. Remember: "Nothing tastes as good as thin feels."

7. Here's an exercise you may have heard of before but never tried. I urge you to try it because the results are fantastic and well worth the embarrassment and discomfort it may cause.

Have someone take full-length pictures of you, from the front, side and back, while you're either in underwear or in a swimsuit. Embarrassed just thinking about doing it? Well, maybe that's a clue that you really need to do this because you're not facing what condition your body's in right now. However, if you really can't face the idea of having someone looking at your aft and taking pictures of it, then consider borrowing a 35mm camera with a delayed timer and take the picture yourself.

You may be in for a shock when the pictures are returned from the developer. Most of us have distorted mental pictures of what our bodies look like—we tend to exaggerate how fat we think we are in some areas of our body, and minimize our measurements in others.

After you've recovered from your feelings of surprise and/or horror about the black-and-white truth of your bodily state, don't hide the pictures! Instead, put them where you'll see them regularly. People who live alone or who have understanding roommates should hang the pictures on the refrigerator or pantry door. Others may decide to put the pictures in a cosmetics or underwear drawer, or in another place they regularly look into. As painful as it may be, these pictures will keep you motivated to lose weight.

8. It's also helpful to stand nude in front of a full-length mirror and take a long, hard look at your body. Use a hand-held mirror to look at your backside. Make a note of what parts of your body you'd like to shape up, and what parts of your body you do like. This is important, because while you want to realistically assess what your body looks like, you also don't want to be overly critical of yourself. Everyone has parts of their looks that they do like, and it's important for you to compliment yourself on these things to keep your spirits up.

9. If you have a picture of yourself at a weight you enjoyed, hang that picture up, too. Try to find a picture from when you were feeling especially good about yourself. This will remind you that you *can* get to your goal when you're feeling discouraged.

10. The first three days of a diet are usually uncomfortable no matter what you do, but once you get past the first day, the next day's easier, and the third day is easier than the second. Mentally cut your Yo-Yo Syndrome Diet down into small steps, taking it one day at a time and concentrating on getting through today. Don't worry about going off your diet tomorrow, because you can only control your eating right now, right this minute. If you feel tempted to overeat, tell yourself, "Right this minute, I won't overeat. I won't overeat from now, 10:25, until one minute from now, 10:26." Then when 10:26 comes along, renegotiate with yourself.

11. Portions really are important! And since Snowball Effect Eaters are so good at fooling themselves about the ever-increasing size of their meals, it's vital that you stay brutally honest with yourself about how much you eat. For you, second helpings aren't even an option for you to consider. When you eat something really tasty, make it last by savoring each bite. But don't go back for more until your next meal.

12. Snowball Effect Eaters must remind themselves of food's chief purpose: nourishment. No matter how good food tastes, there's no reason to eat more than it takes to give you a mild feeling of fullness. Admittedly, however, this is easier written than done. Those who have broken out of the Snowball Effect Eaters' cycle invariably follow these guidelines to avoid eating more than they need:

- Chew slowly, putting your fork down between bites.
- Pay attention to the taste and texture of the food in your mouth. Avoid reading or watching television while you're eating; these distractions take your focus off eating, leaving you unaware of how much you've consumed.
- Pay attention to your body when it signals that it's

full (many people lose touch with this). You've probably heard that it takes about 20 minutes for our brain to register a sense of fullness. A lot of calories can be consumed in those 20 minutes before you even realize how stuffed you feel.

- Remember: this isn't your last meal. Many people eat as if there won't be enough food, so they stuff as much food in their mouths as fast as they can. Relax while you eat.

- As soon as you are mildly full (not stuffed), do something to officially signal an end to the meal, thus stopping your eating. You can do this by putting your napkin (or someone's cigarette butt) on any food left on your plate. This will make the food look unappetizing and reduce the chance that you'll pick at it. If possible, get up and throw the rest of the food on your plate in the garbage disposal. Then brush your teeth and floss (take a toothbrush with you to work and to restaurants), and find something to do to take your mind off eating.

13. Many of my clients have found a good way to stop themselves from craving goodies is to use grotesque mental imagery. One client imagined that the cookies she was craving were made by hideous monsters with oozing sores on their hands. Another said she thought about bugs crawling across the potato chips she was about to eat. This method is drastic, but powerful when your willpower feels low.

14. Dieters need to create a pleasant ambiance during mealtimes. Instead of eating out of a can or saucepan, instead of driving through that fast-food place and eat-ing while you drive, make sure you sit down and eat your meal with attractive dinnerware and silverware. Put on some nice soothing music instead of the upset-ting evening news, and buy some fresh flowers for a centerpiece. A relaxing dining atmosphere will help keep you from gobbling your meals.

15. Along the same lines, it's important to eat your meals at approximately the same time every day. This helps set the healthier eating habits you'll adopt using the Yo-Yo Syndrome Diet.

16. Buy a non-caloric treat you can give yourself the next time you feel like having a "goody." This can mean buying yourself a new record album or a new book by your favorite author and saving it until you have a craving.

17. Don't put off losing weight any longer. There's no better day than today to begin dieting—don't play that old "I'll wait until Monday" routine; you're just fooling yourself anyway. Some people spend their whole lives *planning* and not doing. Don't be like that with your weight—it won't come off on its own. Keep in mind this adage: "If it's going to be, it's up to me."

18. If you're a recreational eater and overeat mainly for the "fun" of it, then add some real entertainment to your life. Call your local parks and recreation depart-ment and see what hobby classes are being offered— and then join one. Other ideas for fun: throw a "low-calorie party," that is, one centered around something other than food (like swimming, conversation or drink-ing low-calorie beverages); rent a comedy movie; go roller-skating with a friend; attend a local theatrical production; take photographs of nature; take on a project such as renovating an old house for resale or rental; or go to an amusement park.

19. Don't keep junk food around the house. If you have some in your refrigerator or pantry now, get rid of it. If this is impractical because of your family members, then make your own shelf in the pantry and the refrigerator. Remember that all foods not on your shelf are off-limits.

20. If you feel as if you're going to eat, go paint your fingernails right away! You can't eat while your nails are wet, and this will give you time to think about why you want to eat. Are you really hungry or just eating out of habit or emotional influences? Men can keep a pair of work gloves nearby to slip on when the "hungries" attack. Bulky gloves make eating difficult and nibbling almost impossible.

21. Visualize yourself in some outfit that you've always wanted to wear but don't feel you're thin enough for—perhaps a leather miniskirt, a bikini, shorts or straight-legged blue jeans. Make the mental image as vivid as possible. The next time you want to overeat, switch off the thoughts about food by replacing them with your mental picture in your "skinny" outfit. Picture the admiring glances you'll get from others and how good you'll feel and how comfortable you'll be in your body. Then ask yourself what you'd rather have, the food now, or the body later.

22. Learn to spot your self-defeating thoughts about dieting. Watch for those seductive little voices that tell you things like, "It won't hurt to go off my diet this week," or "Oh, what's the use, I've blown my diet today anyway."

As soon as you recognize such a thought occurring, think about a little devil-like character and pretend that it is *he* who is telling you to go off your diet. Give the creature a name and a personality; in other words, make this little devil as real for yourself as you can.

Then when you hear the devil's sabotaging voice, tell him (either aloud or in your mind) to "*Stop!* Stop that talk right this instant!" Picture the devil running away in fright. The self-defeating thoughts should disappear along with your mental image of the devil.

23. Try to avoid social activities that revolve around food. Instead of meeting your friends for dinner at a restaurant, why not go to the park or dancing together?

24. Reward yourself every time you have a day in which you don't overeat. Commit to paying yourself a set amount of money for each successful diet day and then *do* it! The rewards of a new diet aren't always apparent in the first few days, and we all need some incentive for sticking with the plan. Spend the money frequently for a present for yourself—something you normally wouldn't buy yourself, such as a pretty wrapped soap, an accessory for your car, a new pair of earrings or a wallet.

Remember, you would have spent the money anyway, but probably on food. Most people tell me they'd spend any amount of money to stop yo-yoing. If this is true of you, then spend the money for non-caloric treats for yourself—believe me, it's a good investment.

25. If you're a late-night snacker, then vow to yourself right now to make the kitchen out-of-bounds after dinner. Have someone else clear the table for you, and bring any beverages you might want in the evening into the room where you'll be.

Your best bet is to take a walk *immediately* after dinner. This gets you out of the house (and away from food), helps relax you (so you're not as apt to Stress Eat), and burns calories. You might even make new friends or become better acquainted with your neighbors on your walks.

26. If you tend to nibble while you're cooking, be sure to keep a glass of water nearby or chew a piece of sugarless gum to stay away from the cheese you're grating or the sauce you're stirring.

It's also helpful to write yourself a large note that reads, *"Nibbled calories do count!"* Put the card above the area where you prepare meals.

27. Notes to yourself really are powerful. Write some encouraging words to yourself and leave them around the house, pack them in your lunch, or hang them on your wall. Cards saying "You can do it!" "You're gonna look great in that bikini," or "Nothing tastes as good as thin feels" can give your diet a shot in the arm.

28. Seasonal Eaters need to keep their wintertime fat pattern in mind as the first leaves of autumn turn. You *can* take control and undo this pattern, beginning with this year. Reread these motivating suggestions every fall and winter, and then *use them!* It's such a wonderful feeling to wear the same size clothes year-round, and not have to think of summer as a time to shed the winter pounds. I wouldn't trade that delicious feeling for any food in the world!

With Chapter 7, we begin Part Two of *The Yo-Yo Syndrome Diet*. Here you'll learn about the eating plan of the Diet as well as how to stay on your Yo-Yo Syndrome Diet despite all the roadblocks that may arise.

Part Two

THE YO-YO
SYNDROME DIET
WEIGHT-LOSS PLAN

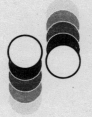

7

The Yo-Yo Syndrome Diet

Step #2 for All Yo-Yo Syndrome Sufferers: Begin the Yo-Yo Syndrome Diet

The Yo-Yo Syndrome Diet is beautiful in its simplicity. That makes it easy to adopt for a lifetime, and easy to remember. It also lacks gimmicks or rigid structure, so you won't tire of it.

If I offered you a rigid diet you would probably react in one of several ways. You might go on the diet and lose weight. But soon you'd tire of the complicated rules of the diet and you'd go back to your old ways of eating and the weight would come back on. Or maybe you'd read the diet and decide that it was impossible for you to follow such strict guidelines. Or perhaps you'd

decide to try the diet and end up resenting the way it
made you feel: controlled by more rigid rules and
boundaries. Nobody likes to be controlled and diets are
extremely controlling by nature.

There's no need for rigid structure to lose weight. In
fact, I don't think permanent weight loss can be
achieved under a rule-laden diet plan. The rules of the
diet become a burden, so the dieter never adopts the
permanent behavioral changes required for lasting
weight loss. And the dieter ends up yo-yoing one more
time.

That's why you'll enjoy the Yo-Yo Syndrome Diet.
Once you stay with it for 30 days, you won't want to
return to your old eating habits. The actual eating plan,
with suggested meals and a shopping list, appears in the
next chapter. In this chapter, you'll begin to familiarize
yourself with the vital information you need to help you
adopt the Diet for a lifetime. First, you must understand
three important guidelines that are fundamental to the
Yo-Yo Syndrome Diet: (1) Always eat three meals a
day; (2) Plan your meals before you eat them; and (3)
Have one helping only.

GUIDELINE 1:
ALWAYS EAT THREE MEALS A DAY

It's important to eat three times per day, although I
understand this concept makes some people anxious.
"But I'll gain weight if I do that!" you may be thinking
right now. I used to believe that if I ate breakfast I'd

gain weight—never realizing that skipping breakfast was keeping me 10 to 55 pounds heavier than I wanted to be. Many of my patients go on the Yo-Yo Syndrome Diet under protest, saying, "It'll make me fat to eat three times a day!" But they try it because they know others are losing weight at my clinics.

These clients are astonished to watch their weight drop without starving, pills or special foods—just as I was myself, when I first discovered the Diet.

If you skip breakfast, you've probably noticed you don't get hungry in the early afternoon. Many people conclude from this that eating breakfast makes them hungrier and therefore makes them eat more food. However, the reason you feel hungry a couple of hours after eating breakfast is that your metabolism—the process that makes you burn calories—has sped up. If you skip breakfast, your metabolism slows down. A slow metabolism makes you fatter because for the rest of the day your body absorbs and uses those calories, and turns them into fat instead of burning them. Yo-Yo Syndrome sufferers already have slow metabolisms, because years of dieting cause permanent slowdowns in metabolism. If you skip breakfast, too, you'll have great difficulty in losing weight permanently.

Breakfast is also important because, without it, your blood sugar level drops, leading to low energy levels and depression. These feelings of tiredness can bring on food binges later in the day as you try to "medicate" the sleepy feelings with food.

Skipping meals does not erase calories from previous binges. The only thing it does is slow down your metabolism so calories take longer to burn. A sluggish metabolism does not "undo" the chocolate cake eaten the day before. Instead, it guarantees that the calories stay in the body longer and turn into body fat quicker.

Skipping meals also sets you up to overeat at your next meal. If you skip breakfast, lunch or dinner, your blood sugar level will drop and you will probably feel light-headed, irritable and weak. Under these conditions, you will be less likely to have the presence of mind to avoid your binge foods at the next meal. When you don't feel well, you are also less likely to *care* whether you lose weight or not.

Make sure you always eat three meals per day, and *never* skip a meal! Some people approach eating in a way I call "creative dieting." In creative dieting, a person uses various rationales for skipping meals, such as: "I ate that big dinner and fattening dessert last night, so I'll skip breakfast this morning." Creative dieters approach eating much like a person who juggles money and floats checks to avoid having a check bounce. The juggling system doesn't work very well with either eating or money because it usually ends up collapsing on itself.

If you're a creative dieter, consider this for a moment: If you knew you had to eat three meals a day, would you be as likely to eat a huge dinner or dessert? Or does your creative approach to dieting give you implied "permission" to binge on fattening foods? If it does, then you have fallen into a common, but erroneous, approach to weight loss.

One final question that creative dieters should ask

themselves is, "If it was a system that worked, would I need to lose weight today?"

GUIDELINE 2: PLAN YOUR MEALS BEFORE YOU EAT THEM

Most Yo-Yo Syndrome sufferers eat in inconsistent, haphazard ways. I know that I used to. I'd wait until five minutes before dinnertime to think about what I was going to eat. I'd go to the grocery store practically every day (which is another hallmark of a Yo-Yo Syndrome sufferer) to shop for that day's meals.

Planning your meals helps you lose weight for two reasons: first, if you plan what you're going to eat, you reduce your chances of overeating whatever is in your refrigerator or pantry. How many times have you come home from work, felt as though you were starving, and impatiently ate whatever was handy? If you plan for this normal reaction in yourself by having dinner ready at an earlier time, you won't have to overeat in the late afternoon.

Second, going to the grocery store for dinner at the last minute increases the likelihood that you'll head for fattening, processed foods. Most people know that shopping on an empty stomach is not a good idea, but do it anyway. In fact, many people overeat before going to the store because they rationalize they're not supposed to shop on an empty stomach.

For this reason, I've included in the next chapter a grocery shopping list for Yo-Yo Syndrome Dieters.

I've had trouble with diets in the past because if I haven't had a particular food in my refrigerator, I'm unable to follow the diet plan for that meal or that day unless I go to the grocery store. It's so much easier to adopt the Diet for a lifetime if you always have your Yo-Yo Syndrome Diet ingredients readily available. Take inventory of your refrigerator and pantry frequently. If you find you're low on your diet foods, stock up before you run out!

GUIDELINE 3: HAVE ONE HELPING ONLY

No matter how tempted you are to go back for another taste, more salad dressing or a second serving, *don't*. Make this a very strict guideline in your mind, especially if you're a Snowball Effect Eater.

The Yo-Yo-Syndrome Diet is a release from the bondage of dieting, as Brenda found out. The dark-haired 42-year-old travel agent was initially apprehensive about the Yo-Yo Syndrome Diet. "It seemed too easy and I didn't trust that it would work at first," she remembered. But Brenda felt she had to try it because her Yo-Yo Syndrome had taken her through three diet clubs and nine weight-loss books.

"This eating program was my last hope," she told me later, after losing 55 pounds. "If it hadn't worked, I was just going to give up and accept being fat for the rest of my life." Imagine Brenda's surprise when she lost 16 pounds the first month of her program!

She's not only lost weight, though, she's also gained confidence and enthusiasm. "I think the greatest thing about the diet is how much more time I have now. I used to spend *so much* time either worrying about my diet and weight, or stuffing my face when I wasn't on a diet. Now that I can eat like 'normal' and still lose weight, I feel so free!"

As with any weight-loss program, it's important to check with your physician before you begin.

OTHER GUIDELINES

Between-Meal Snacks

One of the reasons the Yo-Yo Syndrome Diet works so well is because it's easy to adopt into your lifestyle. Most people, for instance, like to snack between meals, and the Diet readily accommodates this habit by offering you a choice of snacks.

Every day, you can have two of the snacks listed below. If you are someone who normally overeats during the afternoon, then you may want to have both snacks then. On the other hand, you may typically overeat at night while relaxing in front of the television set. If so, then save both snacks for the evening. Of course, you can also opt to have one snack after lunch and then the other one after dinner.

I find it disturbing that a number of recent diet books, especially two written by celebrities, advocate going on periodic eating binges. These so-called controlled binges supposedly consist of forgetting about your diet for one or two days and eating whatever you want—thick steaks, banana splits, chocolate cake . . . in other words, the works!

I don't think these binges are a good idea at all. First, they usually consist of gorging yourself on high-fat, high-sodium, high-cholesterol and just plain unhealthy food. Second, these binges are difficult to stop once they've started. Many people, with the best of intentions, go on one of these "controlled binges" only to find that three months later they've regained 20 or 30 pounds again—which is very discouraging for Yo-Yo Syndrome sufferers.

Third, after one of these binges, there's a hung-over feeling from all the sugar, fat, refined flour and red meat that normally goes along with a binge. Why, I ask you, put yourself through such an ordeal? Instead, adopt a moderate and healthy eating style that is permanent. And find ways other than eating to have fun.

Another word of caution: some people who suffer from the Yo-Yo Syndrome don't know *how* to snack! The well-intentioned snack, for this person, usually starts off with a cracker and the rationalization "it only has ten calories in it." This sets off an appetite for another cracker, but this time topped with cheese because "I have to have protein in my diet." One cracker-with-cheese is followed by another. And another, until the "snack" gains momentum like a rolling snowball and turns into a full-blown binge. The snack becomes an endless food bridge connecting breakfast to lunch to dinner.

If this sounds like you, then you may be someone who cannot snack. In other words, some people have very black-and-white, all-or-nothing ways and cannot do anything in moderation. For these folks, like Binge Eaters, there's no such thing as a "snack" or a small treat. Every time they eat between meals, they keep munching away. To combat this natural tendency to eat endlessly, these people should not eat anything between meals in the first place.

If you cannot keep snacks under control, then you must adopt this guideline: have your snacks from the following list immediately after, or along with, your meals. *Do not* snack between meals.

For those who *can* snack without losing control, here's your list of snack options. You may want to photocopy this list to keep it handy. Pick two snacks to have every day. Don't exceed two, though, or your calorie count will be too high and impede your weight loss.

YO-YO SYNDROME DIET SNACK LIST

- 2 cups popcorn, prepared without oil or butter, seasoned with butter-flavored salt.
- 1 slice whole wheat toast, topped with ½ ounce cream cheese.
- 1 hardboiled egg.
- 1 of the following fruits (portion as specified): 1 medium apple, 1 medium banana, ½ medium cantaloupe, 1 cup cherries, 1 medium grapefruit, ½ papaya, 1 pear, 1 large peach, 1 slice (weighing approximately 7 ounces) of pineapple, 2 cups

strawberries, 2 tangerines, or 1 small slice (weighing approximately 11 ounces) watermelon.

- 1 serving non-fat frozen yogurt (no topping) equalling approximately 100 calories.
- ¼ cup raisins.
- 2 large carrots.
- 2 celery stalks, each spread with ⅓ ounce cream cheese.
- 10 whole wheat, low-salt crackers, plain; or 6 whole wheat, low-salt crackers spread with ½ ounce cream cheese.
- 2 cups sugar-free gelatin.
- 1 serving instant soup. Limit this snack to twice a week, however, as it is fairly high in sodium.
- 1 sugar-free frozen confection (e.g., fudge pops, fruit pops) equalling 100 calories or less. *Note:* read the ingredients label carefully to make sure the product is sugar-free. Some are low in calories, but still contain sugar. Sugar bingers need to be especially aware of this.
- 1 corn tortilla, heated in oven until crisp (don't use oil!), then broken into "taco chips" and served with 1 tablespoon salsa.
- 1 cup unsweetened applesauce, with cinnamon sprinkled on top.
- Lo-Cal Hot Cocoa. This is a delicious drink that tastes high in calories! Try it with breakfast or dinner (but limit yourself to 1 serving or the calories will add up).

1 cup skim milk
1 tablespoon unsweetened baking cocoa
2 packages artificial sweetener

Heat milk in saucepan or microwave. Stir in cocoa and sweetener and mix well.

- Lo–Cal Chocolate Milk Shakes. Ice cream lovers will appreciate diet chocolate milk shakes when they're having cravings. One serving equals one snack.

  1 cup skim milk
  6 ice cubes
  2 packages artificial sweetener
  3 capfuls chocolate extract
  1 capful unsweetened vanilla extract

Put ingredients in blender and mix at medium speed until texture becomes slushy. *Optional:* Add 1 capful cherry, peppermint or coconut extract to the mixture.

- One honey- or fructose-sweetened granola bar 100 calories or under.
- Any snack with 100 or fewer calories. Although your weight loss will be quicker if you avoid high-fat and sugared snacks, you *can* have one of these occasionally on the Yo-Yo Syndrome Diet provided that the snack is not your binge food and that it contains no more than 100 calories.

Beverages

Water. How many of you have heard the old diet adage to drink eight glasses of water a day, and especially to drink water right before a meal? If you're like I used to be, you've heard this, considered it, and then never quite put it into practice. So when I write that an important part of the Yo-Yo Syndrome Diet is to drink those eight glasses of H_2O every day, I know you may ignore me. Yet consider the following facts:

Water is the best defense you have against water retention, bloating and water weight gain. When your diet has too much sodium and salt in it, you begin to retain water and salt in your fat cells and this makes you feel bloated and heavy. Water actually flushes out that salt and retained water.

Water also flushes out waste material your body creates as you lose weight. The fat you'll lose on the Yo-Yo Syndrome Diet will leave your system much faster if you aid it with plenty of water.

Water also helps improve the appearance of your skin. Sometimes dieters get what's known as "dieter's pall," meaning a gaunt, haggard look to their faces. Drinking plenty of water is the best way to combat this. Top models know that water is one of the best beauty secrets you can use.

Water is energizing. The next time you feel lethargic or in an energy slump, reach for a glass of ice water instead of a cup of coffee, and see if you don't feel your energy level pick up. This energizing effect will help keep you away from snacks during those times when you're apt to reach for a candy bar as a pick-me-up.

If possible, try to make your water a special beverage by drinking out of a beautifully cut glass or crystal glass, garnished with a slice of lemon or lime. This will help stop the sense of deprivation that thinking "it's just a glass of water" brings about.

If you don't have ready access to fresh water at work,

then bring in your own! I bring a gallon container to my office every day, so that water is handy at my desk. When water is easy to get and in plain view, I'm less likely to forget or skip my daily water quota.

Soda. Diet sodas can quench that desire for something sweet as well as give you a feeling of fullness that will keep you from snacking. Some of the new diet chocolate soft drinks taste good and help when chocolate cravings begin. A word of caution, however: Yo-Yo Syndrome sufferers, because of their extreme sensitivity to mood-altering chemicals, are especially susceptible to caffeine addiction or abuse. Many of my clients were "hooked' on diet colas containing caffeine and aspartame (marketed under the name NutraSweet) because of the high that they gave them. More on caffeine and NutraSweet brand sweetener appears below.

While diet sodas are excellent drinks for dieters, some people retain water if they drink too many soft drinks. The caramel-colored sodas, in particular, tend to cause water retention. If you drink more than three diet colas per day and you're not happy with your weight loss rate, try cutting back on soft drink consumption to see if this propels weight loss.

Fruit-flavored Sparkling Water. Avoid waters flavored with high-calorie sweeteners such as fructose or corn syrup. Just because the bottle says "all natural" or "no sugar added" doesn't mean that the drink is low-calorie. Also, sparkling water containing fruit juice may add more calories than you anticipated to a meal. In addition, make sure the water is low in sodium, to avoid water retention.

Coffee. Coffee fits into your diet well for two reasons: first, it's low in calories, and second, it satisfies other cravings, particularly cravings for chocolate. Pyrazine, the chemical in chocolate that activates the pleasure center in the brain, is also found in the smell of coffee; if you're dying for chocolate, take a deep whiff of ground coffee or make a pot of coffee and let the smell drift through your home.

Many chocoholics get rid of their cravings by having a cup of chocolate-flavored coffee (giving them a double dose of pyrazine!). Flavored coffee is sold at gourmet food stores, coffee shops and large supermarkets; however, I don't recommend them for several reasons. First, they tend to be expensive; I think, you can make a better mixture yourself by adding unsweetened powdered cocoa and artificial sweetener or cherry, peppermint or vanilla extract to your coffee. (Adding skim milk and artificial sweetener brings out the flavor even more.) Second, many instant coffees that are flavored and presweetened with artificial sweeteners are often high in calories because of extra ingredients such as fats and oils. Third, these mixes are too convenient and lend themselves to binges. At 60 to 90 calories per cup, a binge on these coffee mixes can add up to a lot of calories!

If you prefer cream with your coffee, try to stick to skim milk. Dry creamers are loaded with fat products and are high in calories.

One final point on coffee, particularly chocolate-flavored coffee: be careful not to have too much caffeine. While caffeine creates an energizing feeling, remember that the surge of energy is soon followed by a lull and feelings of lethargy, leading to the desire for more chocolate and caffeine. In addition, the anxiety and nervous energy from stimulant intake is often confused with hunger. So consider having decaf on your coffee break, especially in the afternoon or evening.

Tea. Another hot drink that works well at reducing chocolate cravings is tea. I recommend herbal teas because of their delicate taste, their lack of caffeine, and the relaxing quality of certain herbs such as camomile. Recently, I've found two or three good-tasting brands of carob tea at health food stores. They're not only extremely low in calories, they're also good chocolate substitutes!

If you haven't experimented with the various flavors of tea currently on the market, I urge you to try them. Herb teas, containing no caffeine, are a particularly good antidote for late-night urges to snack. Be sure to try orange-cinnamon (it tastes sweet without sugar), jasmine, carob with spices (good for chocolate cravings) and almond.

Ginger Ale. One of the addictive and mood-affecting chemicals in chocolate, tyramine, is found in large quantities in ginger ale. Drinking a can of diet ginger ale, for this reason, often reduces or eliminates cravings for chocolate.

Alcohol. I recommend that alcohol consumption be limited to white and blush wines (such as white zinfandel) and light beer, to avoid the high amount of calories contained in other forms of liquor. To cut calories even further, try making a low-calorie wine cooler by mixing diet orange or lemon-lime soda with white wine. It's delicious! Just remember that each glass of wine or beer replaces one snack on your daily snack allowance.

On Vitamin and Amino Acid Supplements

The amino acids, especially arginine, ornithine, glutamic acid, tyrosine, phenylalanine and tryptophan, are excellent at reducing cravings for sweets, dairy products and chocolate. Most come in 500-mg tablets or capsules, and I recommend starting with one of each in the morning. (Check with your doctor first and make sure the amino acids are FDA approved.) For convenience, you may want a pre-mixed amino acid tablet or powder that contains all the amino acids listed above (but stay away from mixtures that contain sugar, fructose or corn syrup).

If you feel at all irritable or nervous after starting with this dosage, cut back to 250 mg of tyrosine and phenylalanine (the stimulant amino acids). In addition, if you drink or eat anything containing aspartame (marketed under the brand name NutraSweet), you may not need to take a phenylalanine supplement. This sweetener contains large amounts of phenylalanine, and is one reason that people report mood changes after drinking several diet sodas. Phenylalanine, in moderate amounts, is a stimulant and appetite suppressant. In too great a quantity, however, it leads to mood swings and confusion in some people; cut down if you feel out–of–sorts in any way.

Tryptophan*, the natural sedative amino acid, is good for combating afternoon and evening cravings. Many of my clients crave their binge food most between 3:00 and 4:30 p.m., so I recommend one tryptophan caplet an hour before their cravings usually begin (the chemical takes about an hour to start working). For my patients who have trouble falling asleep, I recommend one to three tryptophan caplets an hour before bedtime and all have reported the same results: a deep, restful sleep that doesn't feel drug–induced. The amount of tryptophan you should take depends on your body weight and sensitivity to chemicals. Start with one caplet and adjust from there. If you don't take enough, you won't feel the effect, but if you take too much, you'll feel groggy the next day.

Amino acids come in two forms, indicated by the letter "L" or "D" in front of the chemical's name (e.g., L-tryptophan). The L indicates a natural form of the amino acid, while a D signifies a synthetic version. L is considered a superior form to D or even the occasional L–D mixtures; therefore, I recommend taking only the L form.

I also recommend vitamin supplements, although I don't think mega doses are always necessary. A vitamin that supplies 100 percent of the minimum daily requirements for all vitamins and minerals is generally suffi-

* As this book was being printed, the FDA issued a warning about L-tryptophan because of reports linking the drug to flu-like symptoms. Accordingly, you should consult a health professional familiar with current research on tryptophan before you use it.

cient; women should take an additional iron and calcium supplement.

Both amino acid and vitamin supplements help keep you feeling good physically and psychologically. When you feel good, you won't be as likely to open the refrigerator looking for some food that will make you feel better.

Step #3 for Binge Eaters:
Abstain from Your Binge Food

For Binge Eaters, the return to compulsive overeating —and weight gain—always begins with one bite of a binge food. Some try to fight their binge food by thinking, "If only I can get thin enough, then I'll be able to eat brownies [or whatever the binge food is] just like a normal person." They believe that weight loss will give them the ability to eat binge foods in moderation. This is the fantasy of every Binge Eater, who unfortunately often has to learn through multiple weight gains and losses that there really is no such thing as one bite of the binge food.

In fact, for most Binge Eaters, even the smallest particle of a binge food can set off a powerful craving for more. So bread bingers must avoid all foods made with refined (and in some cases, whole wheat) flour. This means getting into the habit of checking the ingredients labels of foods and asking lots of questions when ordering at restaurants. Many bread bingers also find they have to abstain from other forms of grains such as oats, rye and cornmeal. The starch portion of their diet is made up with foods that don't trigger binges, such as potatoes, whole corn or rice.

Sugar bingers, too, have to watch for hidden sources of sugar by reading the ingredients of foods they buy. In addition, learn to avoid the other forms of sugar such as glucose, fructose, corn syrup, dextrose, honey and sucrose. If any of these sweeteners triggers binges in you, avoid them as well as sugar.

Salty junk food bingers will need to avoid foods that are salty, fried or crunchy in order to abstain. Again, become very aware of what you're buying at the store or what you're ordering at a restaurant to avoid getting your binge food in hidden forms (more on this in Chapter 10).

For those whose binge foods are crunchy snacks such as potato chips, there are several ways to reduce cravings. First, have on hand crunchy non-caloric items such as frozen diet pops that you can make yourself or buy. Or try chewing sugarless gum to quell between-meal urges to eat. When using gum as a means to reduce cravings, try to choose brands that have NutraSweet brand sweetener because the artificial sweetener sorbitol has a laxative effect and produces gas or intestinal discomfort.

Spicy food bingers will have to avoid the peppery, garlicky, salty and oniony foods that trigger their compulsive overeating episodes. Instead, these Yo-Yo Syndrome sufferers will need to learn to enjoy eating "tamer" versions of their binge food—a subject discussed in Chapters 8 and 10. I've also had some spicy food binger clients who, after they quit smoking cigarettes, learned to better appreciate the non-spicy foods because their taste buds became more sensitive.

Dairy food bingers need to guard against hidden sources of creamy sauces or cheeses. This can require quite an adjustment, as dairy products are found in so many foods. For some Yo-Yo Syndrome sufferers, dairy food binges take the form of overeating *all* dairy products—anything containing milk sets off an eating binge. Others binge only on certain dairy products, such as cheese or ranch-style dressing, and so are able to freely eat dairy products except for the particular one they binge on.

Chocolate bingers must distinguish if they become out of control when eating *all* forms of chocolate, or just chocolate desserts containing refined sugar. The latter type of Binge Eater doesn't need to stop eating chocolate, but instead must switch to unsugared forms of chocolate such as frozen chocolate yogurt sweetened with honey or fructose, chocolate frozen confections sweetened with aspartame (NutraSweet brand sweetener) or chocolate candies made with sorbitol. If you're unsure of your particular brand of chocolate binging, then experiment with these unsugared desserts. Pay careful attention to your reactions—if you feel the urge to voraciously binge, then you'll need to abstain from that form of chocolate.

If you're really afraid that you'll binge on those cookies, nuts, pizza slices or other foods currently in your house, get rid of them! Either throw them away, put them down the garbage disposal, get someone else to eat them or just get as far away from them as you can. Remember, fat on your body is more of a waste than throwing away food. Most Yo-Yo Syndrome sufferers have spent hundreds, maybe thousands, of dollars in efforts to lose weight. They've spent even more money buying binge foods. The point is to not let a sense of false economy keep you from throwing out temptation.

Once you give up your binge food, you'll have more free time and stop obsessing over food. Yes, the first three or four days without your binge food *will* be difficult. You'll miss it. And you may experience negative emotions since your binge food was helping you keep a lid on these feelings. But once you make it past the discomfort of those initial few days, you'll find that your desire for your binge food gradually fades away.

Some days, you'll desperately crave your binge food, but for the most part you'll find that your binge food becomes "out of sight, out of mind." You'll feel in control of yourself and you'll lose weight. And because you won't be yo-yoing or binge/starving anymore, your body will be healthier and you'll feel mentally alert. The swings in your weight, concentration and mood will disappear.

Step #4 for Binge Eaters and Step #3 for All Other Yo-Yo Syndrome Sufferers: Keep Up Your Motivation

After you stick to the Diet (which you'll read more about in the next chapter) for 30 consecutive days you'll find that this new way of eating is automatic. If you eat according to the Diet, you will lose between three and six pounds the first week. Most people continue weight loss at the rate of one to three pounds each week thereafter.

This rate of weight loss is fast enough to satisfy most dieters, while also being slow enough to ensure that the weight loss will be *permanent*. This is important. Sure, I could describe a diet to you that would make eight pounds a week vanish from your body, but how long could you keep up a bland, highly restricted diet without going on an all-out, who-cares-anyway-about-losing-weight eating binge?

The Yo-Yo Syndrome Diet offers you a way to realistically take the weight off and keep it off without getting bored or feeling deprived. On this weight-loss program, you get two snacks and three fairly generous meals *every* day. As long as you stay aware of your emotional, stress-related and motivational issues and don't mix them up with hunger, you shouldn't feel much temptation to break your diet.

However, we all struggle with "the hungries" now and then—this is part of the Yo-Yo Syndrome. If you're like the typical Yo-Yoer, you'll often go on a diet and swear you'll lose weight because an isolated event—perhaps a comment about the size of your stomach or bottom—has made you feel fat. Right at that moment, your motivation to shed the pounds is high! Unfortunately, however, this attitude often fades after one to two weeks of facing another plate of watercress and sliced tomatoes. At that point your thoughts are usually along the lines of, "Who cares about looking good? Just give me some real food!"

To keep your motivation high, it's important to incorporate the guidelines of the Yo-Yo Syndrome Diet into your everyday lifestyle. There is a beginning to the Diet, but no ending, because it's not so much a weight-loss plan as it is a new way of living for you. Once your excess weight comes off, you must shift your attention to keeping it off, a subject discussed further in Chapter 12.

Step #4 for Binge Eaters and #3 for all other Yo-Yo Syndrome sufferers helps you keep your focus on your original goal of losing weight. It's a two-fold simple process that must be incorporated into your daily lifestyle: (1) weigh yourself every morning, and (2) look at your body in a full-length mirror every day after weighing yourself (Snowball Effect Eaters may recognize these suggestions from their list of motivational tips, given in Chapter 6).

WEIGH YOURSELF EVERY MORNING

The first part of this step involves making sure your scale is accurate. If you're not sure, if the scale is ancient, then buy yourself a new one with digital readout (so you're absolutely certain of your exact weight).

Then make this a daily habit: right after awakening and urinating, take off your pajamas and weigh yourself in the nude. Don't drink or eat anything before you weigh yourself, and always keep the scale in the same location in the bathroom as variations in the floor can make your weight erroneously appear to fluctuate.

There is no need to weigh yourself more than once a day. Your weight will naturally increase two to four pounds during the day because of fluid and food intake, so scale readings are most accurate in the morning. By weighing yourself every morning, you get daily feedback about how yesterday's eating has affected today's weight. After a while, you'll notice patterns in your weight, such as a one- to two-pound weight gain after eating food high in sodium the day before.

Don't worry about tiny fluctuations in your weight. Everyone's weight wavers one to two pounds now and then, especially the closer you get to your goal weight (when weight loss slows down to a snail's pace). However, it's vital you guard against dieter's complacency —that attitude of not caring whether you gain weight or not.

If you stop losing weight for more than one week, *or* if your weight loss during the first month of the Diet ever becomes less than one pound a week, *or* if you gain more than two pounds, don't ignore it. Take action right then and go back to carefully weighing and measuring your foods, as will be described in Chapter 8.

LOOK AT YOUR BODY IN A FULL-LENGTH MIRROR EVERY DAY AFTER YOU WEIGH YOURSELF

If you don't already own a full-length mirror (5 to 6 feet long), then buy one right away. Many Yo-Yo Syndrome sufferers fool themselves about their weight gains by looking only at their faces—and not their bodies—in the mirror; or just glancing at their bodies when they get out of the shower; or looking at their bodies full-length only when they're dressed; or looking into a mirror reflection of themselves from the waist (sink-high) up only.

Chapter 6 describes the process of initially rediscovering your body in the mirror in great detail. If you haven't already done so, read the description on page 113—and then do it.

Every day, right after you weigh yourself, take two to three minutes to stand in front of your full-length mirror and look at your naked body from the front and the back.

Spend some time looking at your entire torso: your bottom and thighs. Your stomach and upper arms. All around, front and back, look at your body as if you were seeing it for the first time.

Both of these exercises will help you reaffirm on a daily basis your commitment to losing weight and keeping it off. Make them a habit that you faithfully adhere to, regardless of the circumstances. If you are traveling, ask the hotel staff for a scale when you check in (almost all hotels can oblige this request), or pack your own scale in your suitcase to bring along. If you're staying at a friend's house, ask to borrow his or her scale. Weigh yourself and look at your full-length body every day.

Some Thoughts to Keep in Mind

You'll make losing weight easier on yourself if you incorporate the following time-honored habits into your new lifestyle:

- Try to eat your meals at the same time every day.
- Always eat sitting down. Too often, we'll stand in front of the refrigerator and not realize how much we're consuming, a nibble at a time.
- When you first sit down to your meal, wait two minutes before you begin to eat (the food will still be hot!). This will set the pace for a slower, more relaxed meal and you'll feel more in control of yourself while you're eating.
- Chew your food slowly and put your fork down between bites. I know you've heard that one before, but have you learned to do it yet?
- In the middle of your meal, stop eating for at least two minutes. It's even a better idea to excuse yourself from the table, go to another room and stretch for a while before resuming your meal. This will give your stomach time to tell your brain that it's starting to fill up with food, as well as give you a

moment to change your mind if you were about to overeat.

- Get into the new habit of leaving at least one tablespoon of food on your plate. Cleaning your plate is passé!

- Immediately either throw away your leftovers, freeze them or put the serving dishes in the sink and pour water on them. If you have trouble even getting into the kitchen without eating the leftovers, then have someone else clear the table for you.

- The minute you think of going off your diet, distract yourself by doing something involving physical activity. If you're sitting at your desk, take a walk down the hall (staying clear of the cafeteria and vending machines, of course) or stand up and stretch. If you're home, get out of the house and take a pleasant walk, ride a bike or go to the gym. These activities not only distract you from eating, they also focus you on your goal of losing weight. It makes little sense, after going to the trouble of exercising, to undo all that hard work with a high-calorie meal. Besides, exercise has a great way of reducing the appetite. In addition, exercising on a regular basis helps you to burn more calories by increasing the rate of your metabolism.

- When you're hungry, drink a non-caloric beverage, such as water, tea or a diet soft drink, and put it in a beautiful glass, garnished with a slice of lemon. In this way, you'll feel full because of the liquid and you'll also feel less deprived if you make the drink

look special. I've found, also, that late-night cravings really disappear when I have a hot drink such
as herbal tea.

- Here's another tip for when you feel an irresistible
urge to eat between meals: brush your teeth, floss
them and then gargle. Your mouth will feel so
clean that the desire for food will vanish. Besides,
you won't want to dirty your teeth after cleaning
them.

- You'll find that you'll feel more full after a meal if
you focus your attention on eating. Many people
read, watch television, work or drive while they
eat, and they can't imagine sitting down to a meal
and just eating. If your attention is diverted away
from eating because of a book or TV, you may not
be aware of how much you're eating, or when you
are full.

    If you can break this habit, however, you'll find
that you feel more satisfied after meals because of
the increased awareness of the taste and feeling of
the food in your mouth. Try to appreciate all the
sensations of eating at your meals. What colors are
in the foods? What smells? How about the texture
of the food in your mouth—how does it feel? What
does your stomach feel like when you're full? Paying attention to questions like these will help keep
you from overeating.

- Snowball Effect Eaters should avoid "all you can
eat" restaurants for at least the first month of their
diet. These places just prey on Snowball Effect
Eaters' difficulties with portion control and their

normal desire to get their money's worth of food. The endless buffets at all-you-can-eat restaurants offer such a variety of textures and tastes that it's tempting to eat just a little bit of everything. This usually results in plates stuffed with food, however, and may send you back for second helpings of that food you especially enjoyed. So if you decide to try an all-you-can-eat place, after you've been on the Diet for at least a month, stick to the following plan:

Decide to eat only six items from the buffet. For instance, two different kinds of meat, two salads and two side dishes. Remember the Diet Plan principle of *one serving only*. No matter how much you're tempted to get "just a little bit more" food, it's important you don't. (This plan also works well for other kinds of gatherings at which a lot of food is offered, such as Thanksgiving dinners, weddings, parties, company picnics and family gatherings.)

- It's also important to stop thinking about eating as recreation. For many Snowball Effect Eaters and Stress Eaters, eating is the only "fun" in their life. No wonder, then, it's such a struggle to give up! Often, people who feel this way are overworked and over-responsible and don't make room in their lives for non-competitive fun and relaxation. They have "fun" by curling up with a bowl of ice cream or a bag of potato chips. Eating forces them to momentarily relax, so they pair food with pleasure.

If this sounds like you, it's important to ask

yourself: was it *really* fun to overeat and have all those unpleasant sensations that go along with it? Remember feeling fat, sluggish, out of control and angry at yourself for eating so much? Is there a better way to really have fun?

- Just as many Yo-Yo Syndrome sufferers use food as a way of having "fun," many use food when they're feeling lonely. Self-Esteem Eaters and Emotion Eaters need to stop thinking about food as companionship. True, food won't say mean things or reject you in the way that humans sometimes do, but it's also a poor substitute for true intimacy with another person.

  If you have used food as a "friend," you will probably experience some feelings of grief (such as anger or depression) after you give up compulsive overeating. The best remedy for this process is to just go ahead and face the feelings. Chapter 3 describes more specific ways to handle upsetting feelings that occur as you let go of your old ways of eating, so you may want to reread that chapter to help you face the griefwork.

- Because Emotion Eaters use food to "stuff down" their uncomfortable emotions, they may find that they're particularly emotionally vulnerable during the first two weeks of the eating plan. Food no longer anesthetizes emotions in the Yo-Yo Syndrome Diet, so feelings seep out into the open. For this reason, there's usually a great desire to eat as soon as one of those uncomfortable emotions creeps into awareness.

Feelings such as anger, disappointment, insecurity and loneliness are often confused with hunger because we're so used to reaching for food the moment these emotions begin to surface. In addition, many people feel irritable or slightly depressed during the first three days of their diet and mistakenly think these feelings mean they're either malnourished or starving to death. This frightening thought sends many people to the refrigerator. What they don't realize, however, is that their previous overeating habits were masking the angry or depressing feelings that were always there. Now that they're not overeating, these emotions are fully—and often uncomfortably—felt.

The next time you feel like overeating, ask yourself: what is the *emotion* I'm trying to run away from? Stay out of the kitchen and promise yourself not to eat for the next 15 minutes while you think about your feelings. Chances are good that at the end of the 15 minutes, the urge to eat will have passed.

If you want to eat when you're really not hungry, you may actually be trying to escape an unpleasant feeling. Often, just by admitting to yourself you're feeling a certain way (i.e., sad, guilty, resentful, etc.), you can diffuse the feeling before it leads to overeating.

If you're unsure what it is you're feeling, try writing down the thoughts you have about the day's events. Often, this brainstorming with yourself will uncover some anger or anxiety. Just pinpointing the source of your feelings will bring about a sense of relief, and focusing on your thoughts and emotions will likely reduce your "hunger."

- Sometimes food cravings occur because we're putting off doing some unpleasant task such as writing that letter, filling out those loan papers, making that unpleasant phone call, or cleaning that room. The next time you're "hungry," ask yourself if you're actually avoiding doing something else. If so, perhaps there's some small step you can take right now toward accomplishing the dreaded task. For instance, getting the paper and pens ready, getting the phone number out, or assembling the cleaning supplies. The task won't feel so overwhelming if you break it down into small, easy-to-accomplish steps. On the other hand, maybe the task could be delegated to someone else.

If you feel your motivation level wavering or falling at any time, be sure to reread the section on Step #1 for Snowball Effect Eaters in Chapter 6. It contains suggestions to help spur you on toward your goal of a slim body for a lifetime.

8

Your Eating Plan

THIS CHAPTER thoroughly explains the Yo-Yo Syndrome Diet and outlines some sample meals that you can choose from.

The meals in this chapter do not contain sugar and are mostly low in fat and cholesterol and high in fiber. While this is not a strict requirement of the Diet, it is a good idea for health and caloric reasons to eat foods that are sugar-free and low in fat.

In particular, fat is a major contributor to the calories in most meals because it contains five more calories per gram than either protein or carbohydrates. Fat also is converted to body fat almost four times faster than carbohydrates. So it makes sense to reduce fat as much as you can from your diet by:

- Avoiding fast foods such as hamburgers, fried chicken, french fries and deep-fried foods.
- Limiting red meat consumption to a maximum of one serving per week.
- Removing the skin from chicken.
- Buying only lean cuts of meat.
- Using small portions of fatty sauces and dressings containing butter.
- Learning what foods are high in fat (for instance, nuts, salty junk foods, processed lunch meats, beans and avocados) and cutting down on them.
- Using the non-fat or low-fat versions of foods such as cottage cheese, milk, cheese or yogurt.
- Using as little oil, butter or margarine in cooking as possible.

When grocery shopping, be sure to read labels carefully so you'll know how much fat foods contain. Try to keep the amount of fat in your daily diet to 20 percent or less of your total food consumption and you'll cut a lot of calories automatically. It will, however, take about a month to adjust to lowered amounts of fat in your diet. This is because high-fat foods make you feel full for a long time since they are difficult to digest and stay in the stomach longer than other, more easily digestible foods. But don't despair—after approximately 30 days your stomach, and you, will learn to be satisfied with a low-fat diet.

When reading labels, Binge Eaters need to watch for hidden binge foods in the ingredients. Bread bingers, for instance, should avoid flour in the ingredients of processed foods, soups and frozen dinners. Sugar bingers need to remember to watch for fructose, glucose, sucrose, corn syrup and in some cases honey (depending on whether this triggers a binge or not).

As mentioned in Chapter 7, it is very important to have your Yo-Yo Syndrome Diet foods on hand in your refrigerator or pantry to avoid last-minute trips to the store, and to avoid overeating whatever's handy. To help out, I've outlined what you might want to buy each week at the grocery store to keep your kitchen well-stocked. This list, of course, is intended as an example, so don't feel you must follow it precisely. You can, however, follow it exactly if you're unsure of how to organize your new diet around your life. (Note: Binge Eaters need to avoid any items containing their binge food that may be on this list.)

Either bring this book to the grocery store with you or copy the list so you won't forget an important item. This list covers enough food for one person for one to two weeks on the Yo-Yo Syndrome Diet; if you're shopping for other people who'll be dieting with you, multiply the items accordingly. I've organized the list into sections that are normally found in a grocery store.

YO-YO SYNDROME DIET GROCERY LIST

Produce Section
2 large apples
2 medium bananas
2 large oranges

1 package celery
1 large head iceberg or greenleaf lettuce
2 medium brown onions
1 large ripe tomato
3 large russet potatoes
4 large carrots
1 package broccoli
4 to 6 mushrooms
1 eggplant
1 clove garlic

Shelf-Food Section
3 packages sugar-free gelatin
3 cans (8 ounces each) unsugared fruit packed in juice (sliced peaches, crushed pineapple, fruit cocktail)
2 cans (6½ ounces each) tuna fish packed in water
1 box unsugared cereal such as Kellogg's Nutri-Grain or Ralston Sunflakes
1 box (2 servings) instant soup mix
1 box (any size) wild rice
1 box (medium size) white rice
1 pound coffee
2 boxes herb tea

Bakery
1 loaf whole wheat bread
1 package whole wheat muffins or bagels

Spices and Condiments
ground cinammon
1 bottle chocolate extract

1 package artificial sweetener

1 jar dijon mustard

1 jar low-fat mayonnaise

1 jar salt-free seasoning mixture (such as Spike or Mrs. Dash)

1 jar butter-flavored salt

1 can non-stick cooking spray (such as Pam)

Optional:

ground nutmeg

ground allspice

1 bottle unsweetened vanilla extract

1 bottle peppermint, coconut or cherry extract

1 bottle Cajun seasoning mix

1 container unsweetened Hershey's cocoa powder

Dairy Case

1 large (32-ounce) carton low-fat cottage cheese

1 large (32-ounce) carton plain non-fat yogurt

½ gallon skim milk

1 dozen medium eggs

1 package low-calorie margarine

Deli Section

1 small package plain cream cheese

1 package of a low-fat variety of cheese, such as mozzarella, low-calorie american or monterey jack

Meat Section

4 pounds chicken breast

1 pound lean round steak

2 medium rainbow trout

½ pound bay scallops
1 pound red snapper
1 cornish game hen

Frozen Foods
1 package frozen unsugared strawberries
1 package frozen unsugared blueberries
3 "light" (300-calorie or less) frozen dinners
1 package sugar-free frozen confections
(fruit pops or fudge pops)

Beverages
4 gallons drinking water
2 bottles (2-liter) diet soda

Non-Food
Small food scale
1- or 2-cup glass measuring cup
1 set measuring spoons
1 shallow glass pan

And Finally, for You
1 slick, glossy high-fashion magazine such as
Glamour, Gentleman's Quarterly or *Mademoiselle* to
inspire you
1 bouquet fresh flowers to add a special ambiance to
your dining area
1 bottle or box of bubble bath, to treat yourself
(especially on nights when you're apt to overeat)

Variety + Simplicity = Dieting Success

Here's a review of the three guidelines discussed in Chapter 7, to keep in mind when planning your menus:

1. Eat three meals per day.
2. Plan your meals before you eat them.
3. Have one serving only.

Chose your meals from the list starting on page 174. Many people like to find one or two breakfast and lunch meals they enjoy and feel comfortable with, and then stick with these. If you like the "safe" feeling a breakfast and lunch routine affords you, then choose one or two of these meals each, and then plan on using them for a while. It's important, though, for the long-term success of any diet, that you vary your meals as often as you can. Snowball Effect Eaters are especially prone to "dieting burnout," so they need to follow the suggestions for variation outlined below.

Dinners should have a little more variety than the two other meals of the day. Again, choose your meals from the list beginning on page 120. And in Chapters 10 and 11, you'll learn how to take your Yo-Yo Syndrome Diet out into the "real world" of restaurants, parties, work, vacations and holidays and still manage to lose weight and keep it off.

Initially, you should weigh and measure your food to learn what a portion looks like. After one month on the diet, you should be able to "eyeball" what constitutes a portion and stop measuring, unless you eat something new. I firmly believe that diets which ask you to continually weigh and measure are set-ups for failure and weight gain, because they cause you to obsess about eating. The Yo-Yo Syndrome Diet's aim, on the other hand, is to reduce or remove your obsession with food and help you to seek other less fattening ways to feel fulfilled.

Follow the meal suggestions for the first month, or stick to them longer if you like. However, as mentioned before, variety is important in order to maintain your motivation when you adopt a diet. The key to lifelong weight loss and maintenance is *lifelong changes in eating behavior*. The Yo-Yo Syndrome Diet helps you construct your own balanced eating plan and adopt low-calorie eating habits for the rest of your life.

This means becoming aware of balancing your meals, by following these guidelines every day in your diet:

Breakfast consists of one serving (serving sizes are explained below) from the fruit group, one serving from the dairy group and one serving from the starch group.

Lunch includes one serving from the fruits and vegetables group and one serving from the dairy group. In addition, you may choose to have one serving from the meat group and one serving from the starch group. As explained below, men will be eating additional servings of meat and starch because of their higher caloric needs.

Dinner should include one serving from the vegetables group, one serving from the dairy group and one serving from the starch group. If you didn't have meat for breakfast or lunch, you may choose to have one serving for dinner.

To keep the Diet simple and easy-to-use, many people choose to have meat at dinner only and make their breakfasts and lunches consist of foods from the fruits, vegetables, starch and dairy groups. Other successful Yo-Yo Syndrome Dieters find that having meat at any *one* meal is an easy way to limit consumption; if they have meat for lunch, for instance, then they have a vegetarian dinner. To simplify the Diet and to reduce fat and calorie intake, you should limit your meat consumption to once a day, and eat red meat (beef, lamb and pork) only once a week. Red meat, eaten to excess, is very high in fat and calories! Ounce for ounce, you'll be able to eat more meat with your meal if you choose low-fat poultry or fish instead of beef or pork.

The Yo-Yo Syndrome Diet evenly distributes the number of calories consumed throughout the day so that your body can operate at maximum efficiency from morning until evening. In addition, this calorie distribution will mitigate pangs of hunger. Each meal is approximately 300 calories and each of your two snacks equals 100 calories. Here is the easy-to-remember plan:

YO-YO SYNDROME DIET MEAL OUTLINE FOR WOMEN

Breakfast:
1 dairy serving, 100 calories
1 fruit serving, 100 calories
1 starch serving, 100 calories

Lunch:
1 dairy serving, 100 calories
1 fruit *or* vegetable serving, 50–100 calories
1 starch serving, 100 calories

Snack:
1 snack from list on pages 131–133, 100 calories

Dinner:
½ dairy serving, 50 calories
1 vegetable serving, 50 calories
1 starch serving, 100 calories
Plus:
1 meat serving (which you can eat at either breakfast, lunch or dinner or equally divide between two meals), 200 calories

Snack:
1 snack from list on pages 131–133, 100 calories
TOTAL: 1200 calories

This brings your daily calorie intake to approximately 1200 calories, with a variation of 100 calories in either direction. This range of calorie intake, from 1100 to 1300, is optimum for most Yo-Yo Syndrome sufferers. The point of the Diet is not to become obsessed with calorie counting, but to trust that if you stay in the range of 1100 to 1300 calories a day and eat a balanced diet, you'll lose weight with a minimum of confusion, headaches and work.

For men, the Diet is similar, with the addition of 300 extra calories derived from the meat and starch groups, as shown below:

YO-YO SYNDROME DIET MEAL OUTLINE <u>FOR MEN</u>

Breakfast:
1 dairy serving, 100 calories
1 fruit serving, 100 calories
1 starch serving, 100 calories

Lunch:
1 dairy serving, 100 calories
1 fruit *or* vegetable serving, 50–100 calories
1 starch serving, 100 calories

Snack:
1 snack from list on pages 131–133, 100 calories

Dinner:
½ dairy serving, 50 calories
1 vegetable serving, 50 calories
2 starch servings, 200 calories
Plus:
2 meat servings (which you can have at either breakfast, lunch or dinner or equally divide between two meals), 400 calories

Snack:
1 snack from list on pages 131–133, 100 calories
TOTAL: 1500 calories

All Yo-Yo Syndrome Dieters should choose their beverages from the list outlined in Chapter 7. In general, try to have non-caloric drinks such as sugar-free soda, water, tea or coffee. If you have one or two alcoholic beverages with dinner, then you must compensate for the added calories by skipping your evening snack.

Like alcoholic drinks, condiments add calories, so they should be limited to those on this list:

lemon juice
low-calorie margarine
mustard
reduced calorie salad dressings (2 to 3 tablespoons)
spices

Weight loss for both men and women using the Yo-Yo Syndrome Diet will be steady instead of rushed; in other words, you'll lose weight that will stay off permanently. And that's the point of this diet, after all! You've lost weight countless times on ridiculous fad plans that resulted in rapid drops in weight through eating plans that couldn't be incorporated into your lifestyle. How long can *anyone* be expected to eat grapefruit only, protein only, or complicated food combinations without saying, "Forget it! It's just not worth the trouble and monotony!" You've dropped weight fast, only to gain it back again. This time, plan on losing your weight at a comfortable rate. Plan, also, on keeping it off for good.

After you've reached your goal weight (which you

will—remember to think positive!), you'll be adding a few more calories to your daily total in such a way that you'll maintain your attractive new figure. This maintenance plan is detailed in Chapter 12.

Your Food Group Selections

There was a time in diet book history when carbohydrates—that is, breads and starches—were considered the big, bad foods to avoid at all costs. Diets during the 1960s and 70s largely consisted of high-fat, high-protein and low-carbohydrate menus. These fad diets, we fortunately know now, were both dangerous and unrealistic in terms of promoting permanent weight loss. Nutritionists today know that starches such as rice, pasta, whole grains and potatoes are some of the best tools a dieter has, because they contain almost no fat, are high in fiber (which is important in reducing the risk of certain types of cancer), low in calories, and contain important vitamins and minerals. Starches cause trouble only if they're smothered with high-sodium seasonings, high-fat dairy products or fatty meat sauces.

Keeping this in mind, the list below shows what a serving of each food group consists of. Since different brands have different calorie counts, please keep in mind that these serving descriptions are generalizations. It's important for you to check the calorie count of the foods you buy, whenever possible, and keep the calorie count of all servings to 100 calories. For meat, the servings should always be kept under 200 calories. Use this list when planning your week's menus (remember Guideline 2!):

DAIRY GROUP

1 cup (8 ounces) skim or low-fat milk

1 cup (8 ounces) buttermilk

1 whole egg, medium

1 ounce plain low-fat cream cheese

1 cup plain non-fat yogurt

½ cup low-fat cottage cheese

1 ounce low-fat cheese, such as monterey jack, mozzarella, swiss, brick, camembert, low-calorie american

2 tablespoons low-calorie margarine

4 tablespoons low-fat sour cream

3 tablespoons low-fat mayonnaise

Avoid: high-fat cheeses such as cheddar; eggnog, chocolate milk made with sugar; ice cream; pre-sweetened yogurt or yogurt drink (too high in calories per portion); whole milk and butter

FRUITS AND VEGETABLES

Fruits
1 large apple
6 medium apricots
1 medium banana

1 cup berries, such as blackberries, boysenberries, raspberries, strawberries, or blueberries

½ medium cantaloupe

1 cup cherries

1 grapefruit

2 cups grapes

2 medium guavas

½ honeydew melon

½ mango

1 large orange

½ papaya

1 large peach

1 pear

1 cup pineapple

3 small plums

2 tangerines

1 small wedge watermelon (approximately 11 ounces)

Avoid: avocados (they're high in fat and calories); fruits dried with sugar (dates, figs, banana chips); and canned or frozen fruit packed in sugar (a.k.a. syrup)

*Vegetables**

1 artichoke

1 cup cooked asparagus spears

2 cups bean sprouts

1 cup beets

---

* All weights refer to weight before cooking.

½ pound broccoli
10 to 12 brussels sprouts
2 cups red or green raw cabbage
2 medium carrots, or 1 large carrot
1 pound cauliflower
5 stalks celery
½ pound eggplant
¼ pound or 1½ cups cooked green beans
20 leaves lettuce, iceberg or greenleaf
20 small fresh or cooked mushrooms
1 medium brown onion
½ cup green peas
20 raw radishes
½ pound spinach
2 medium or 1 large tomato

Avoid: creamed corn; canned or frozen vegetables processed with brine (salt water), butter or cheese sauce

STARCH GROUP

1 slice whole wheat toast
1 whole wheat muffin (approximately 1½ ounces)
1 whole wheat bagel
1 corn tortilla
½ large corn muffin (approximately 1½ ounces)
1 ounce unsugared cereal
10 whole wheat crackers
½ cup cooked pasta (noodles, macaroni, spaghetti)

½ cup white cooked rice

½ cup brown or wild cooked rice

½ cup beans, soaked without sugar (such as pinto, garbanzo and lima beans and split peas)

2 cups popcorn, cooked without oil or butter

1 ear corn on the cob

½ cup canned corn, rinsed to remove salt

1 medium baked russet potato, (3½ ounces), or ½ large (over 5 ounces)

1 medium boiled or baked new (red) potato

squash (all are cooked weights): ½ medium acorn, ¾ cup butternut, 2 cups zucchini, 2 cups summer, ¾ cup winter

½ medium (3 to 4 ounces) sweet potato, baked without sweeteners

½ cup yams, baked without sweeteners

Avoid: breads made with sugar (such as date bread or banana bread); breads made with refined flour; processed baked beans (they contain a lot of sugar); refried beans made with lard (have the vegetarian style only); boxes of rice or noodles containing seasoning mixes (these have too much salt in them!); candied sweet potatoes or yams

MEATS*

Poultry:

3½ ounces chicken, skinned, bone-out
(approximately 1 breast, thigh or drumstick, or
2 wings)

3½ ounces duck, skinned, bone out

3½ ounces white turkey meat, skinned, bone-out

½ cornish game hen

Fish and Seafood

¼ pound of any of the following: bonito, flounder,
salmon, rainbow trout

⅓ pound of any of the following: bluefish, cod,
haddock, halibut, swordfish

½ pound fillets of any of the following: white
freshwater perch, pike, red snapper, sole

½ pound lobster meat

⅓ pound crabmeat

⅓ pound bay scallops

⅓ pound shrimp

6½ ounces tuna packed in water

Beef

2 ounces of the following steaks (without bone):
chuck, club or ribeye

---

* Always cook your meat by boiling, baking, broasting, roasting, microwaving or barbecuing. Never fry! Limit consumption of red meats to once a week or less. All weights refer to weight after cooking.

3 ounces of the following bone-in steaks (weight includes bone): porterhouse or T-bone

3 ounces of the following steaks (lean cuts): blade, flank, round or sirloin

3 ounce rump roast

3 ounces lean (22 percent or less fat) hamburger

Pork

5 slices bacon, grease absorbed with paper towels

2 ounces canadian bacon (approximately 2 slices)

2 ounces lean ham

2 ounces pork, blade, loin or rib (lean cuts, approximately 1 piece)

4 links sausage

Lamb

4 ounces lean leg meat

3 ounces lean loin chops (approximately 2 chops)

3½ ounces lean rib chops (approximately 2 chops)

Liver★

3 ounces beef

2¾ ounces lamb

Veal

3 ounces arm steak

2½ ounces lean cutlet

3½ ounces lean loin chop

★ Limit consumption of liver to twice a month, as it is extremely high in cholesterol.

Miscellaneous Meats
3½ ounces rabbit
4½ ounces venison

Avoid: highly marbled cuts of beef; chicken skin; hamburger containing over 22 percent fat; processed lunch meats (high in salt and fat); canned corned beef hash; sandwich spreads; processed turkey breast (high in salt); ground turkey meat containing over 22 percent fat; breaded fish patties or sticks; chicken nuggets; sausages such as salami, hot dogs and pepperoni

Sample Meals and Recipes

Listed below are sample meals and recipes that all Yo-Yo Syndrome Dieters can follow. Binge Eaters should look for the following symbols next to each meal in order to avoid their binge foods.

Binge Food Symbols:

B—Breads/Grains
D—Dairy Products
C—Cheese
S—Spicy Meals

You can eat any food that doesn't contain your binge food, and many recipes are flexible so that you can delete the ingredients you binge on.

An asterisk (★) appearing next to an item means that cooking instructions are in the recipe section at the end of this chapter.

BREAKFAST

Breakfast A:

D   ½ cup low-fat cottage cheese, topped with one serving of fruit.

B, D   1 piece whole wheat toast, spread with 1 tablespoon low-calorie margarine.

Breakfast B:

D   Omelette, made with 1 medium or 2 small eggs. Cook in non-stick frying pan to avoid using butter, or use cooking spray. Add chopped scallions (green onions) or mushrooms for extra flavor.

C   Add ½ ounce (approx. 2 slices) low-fat cheese such as mozzarella or monterey jack to the omelette.

B   1 piece whole wheat toast, spread with 1 ounce crushed fresh fruit such as strawberries or blueberries.

Breakfast C:

B, D   1 ounce unsugared cereal (check the ingredients label very carefully for sugar; almost all brands have sugar in them), with ½ cup low-fat or non-fat milk.

Top the cereal with one of the following: 1 medium sliced banana, 1 cup sliced strawberries, 1 cup blueberries *or* 1 cup boysenberries.

Breakfast D:

B, D   1 piece whole wheat toast, with ½ tablespoon low-calorie margarine *or* artificially sweetened jam (available in the diet section of your supermarket).

D   1 egg, cooked over easy or sunny-side up, prepared in non-stick pan or with cooking spray.

1 large orange.

Breakfast E:

*Cooked Fruit with Cinnamon.

D   1 cup low-fat or non-fat milk.

B, D   1 whole wheat muffin, spread with ½ tablespoon low-calorie margarine.

Breakfast F:

2 ounces lean beef, turkey or ham. Heat either in microwave or in non-stick frying pan with ½ teaspoon of low-calorie margarine.

C   You can vary this by melting ½ ounce cheese on top of the meat.

B   Serve over 1 piece whole wheat toast.
½ medium cantaloupe.

Breakfast G:

D   1 cup plain non-fat yogurt, mixed with ½ can sliced peaches packed in juice (no sugar), ½ teaspoon cinnamon, artificial sweetener to taste and ½ teaspoon vanilla extract. Stir well.

B, C   1 whole wheat bagel, spread with ¼ tablespoon cream cheese.

LUNCH

Lunch A:

D, S   ★Cold Chicken Curry Salad.

B   ½ cup cooked brown or wild rice.

Lunch B:

D   ★Tuna Salad on bed of lettuce, or

B, D   Tuna Salad sandwich.

Lunch C:

   C   *Chef's Salad.

   B   10 whole wheat crackers.

Lunch D:

  B, D   ½ cup low-fat cottage cheese with 1 serving fresh fruit or 8 ounces canned fruit, packed in own juice.

  B, D   ½ corn muffin, spread with 1 tablespoon low-calorie margarine.

Lunch E:

   B   *Chicken Vegetable Soup.

   D   1 cup non-fat or low-fat milk.

Lunch F:

C, D, S *Chicken Taco Salad.

Lunch G:

B, D, G *Stuffed Baked Potato.

Lunch H:

   B   1 package instant noodle soup.

           1 serving fresh fruit.

   C   1 ounce sliced swiss cheese.

Lunch I:

           1 frozen "light" (300-calorie or less) meal.

DINNER

Dinner A:

        ★Chinese Stir-Fry (with chicken or beef).

B   steamed rice.

D   4-ounce cup of non-fat or low-fat milk.

Dinner B:

B   ★Baked Cornish Game Hen with Wild Rice.

C   steamed mixed vegetables with melted cheese.

Dinner C:

C, S ★Eggplant Mozzarella.

        dinner salad.

B   whole wheat roll.

Dinner D:

        ★Baked Trout.

D   ★Sautéed Zucchini and Baby Carrots.

B   ½ baked potato.

Dinner E:

B, C, D, S ★Spanish-Style Chicken and Rice.

Dinner F:

B   ★Teriyaki Beef and Broccoli with Rice.

D   4-ounce cup of non-fat or low-fat milk.

Dinner G:

           *Barbecued Chicken Shish Kebabs.

B, D   Corn on the cob with low-calorie margarine.

Dinner H:

           1 frozen "light" (300-calorie or less) prepared dinner.

Dinner I:

           *Sautéed Scallops.

B   steamed rice.

C   steamed broccoli with melted cheese.

Dinner J:

S   *Cajun Snapper.

B   whole wheat buns.

           asparagus tips.

RECIPES

Listed on the following pages are recipes for the above meals. Two asterisks signal you to cut the spices in half if you binge on spicy meals.

Cooked Fruit with Cinnamon ✍

1 serving sliced fresh, frozen or canned (unsugared)
peaches or apples
4 tablespoons water
1 teaspoon cinnamon
½ teaspoon nutmeg
¼ teaspoon allspice

Cook fruit, water and spices over medium heat, stirring often until fruit feels tender when pierced by fork. (Canned and frozen fruits tend to cook much faster than fresh fruit.) *Microwave instructions:* place fruit, water and spices in microwave-safe cookware and cover with plastic wrap. Make 1 or 2 holes in wrap to allow steam to escape. Cook on high for 3 minutes. Allow to sit for 2 minutes, then stir. Cook for 2 more minutes on high (4 minutes for fresh fruit), and serve. *(Serves one)* ✍

Cold Chicken Curry Salad ❧

5 tablespoons plain non-fat yogurt
1 tablespoon low-fat mayonnaise
½ teaspoon curry powder★★
¼ teaspoon onion salt★★
1 tablespoon soy sauce★★
1½ cups chicken, cooked and cubed
1 red apple, peeled and cut into small cubes
4 stalks celery, cut into thin slices
Optional *(delete if you binge on these foods):*
2 tablespoons raisins
2 tablespoons slivered almonds
2 tablespoons coconut, grated and unsugared

Mix yogurt, mayonnaise, curry powder, onion salt and
soy sauce well. Fold mixture into chicken in a large
bowl and carefully add apple cubes and celery. Add
raisins, almonds or coconut if desired. Serve over lettuce leaves. *(Serves two)*   ❧

Tuna Salad ❧

3 tablespoons low-fat mayonnaise
3 tablespoons plain non-fat yogurt
1 tablespoon dijon mustard
¼ onion, peeled and diced
¼ cup diced celery
1 small dill pickle, diced
1 can (6½ ounces) water-packed tuna,
thoroughly drained

In a large bowl, mix mayonnaise, yogurt and mustard well. Add onion, celery and pickle. Fold in tuna until mixture is completely blended.

Serving suggestions: serve on bed of lettuce, or in hollow of scooped-out ripe tomato. Unless your binge food is bread, you may also want to use this tuna salad to make delicious tuna sandwiches. *(Serves two)* ❧

Chef's Salad ❧

2 cups torn or shredded iceberg lettuce
½ carrot
2 ounces (2 slices) turkey or chicken
1 ounce swiss, monterey jack, low-calorie american or
mozzarella cheese
low-calorie salad dressing

Place lettuce in large serving bowl. Use cheese grater to grate carrot; garnish top of lettuce. Cut meat and cheese into thin strips and arrange on top of lettuce and carrot. Pour 3 to 4 tablespoons of salad dressing over entire salad. *(Serves two)*   🍃

Chicken Vegetable Soup 🍃

2 chicken breasts, skin and fat removed
1 can (10¼ ounces) chicken broth
2 cans water
2 carrots, diced
¼ onion, peeled and diced
1 medium russet potato, peeled and cubed
2 stalks celery, diced

Cook chicken, chicken broth, water and carrots over medium-high heat until boiling. With large spoon, skim off chicken fat. Simmer soup in covered pot over low heat for one-half hour, stirring often. Add onion, potato and celery and cook for an additional one-half hour. *(Serves two)*   🍃

Chicken Taco Salad 🦃

3 chicken breasts, skin and fat removed
1 cup water
½ brown onion, peeled and diced★★
2 tablespoons diced green chiles★★
3 tablespoons salsa★★
4 cups shredded iceberg lettuce
1 tomato, cubed or diced
2 scallions (green onions), diced
Optional *(delete if you binge on these foods):*
1 cup shredded monterey jack cheese
2 tablespoons low-fat sour cream (or plain low-fat
yogurt)
1 corn tortilla for Home-Style Tortilla Chips

Shred chicken into bite-sized pieces. Pour water into frying pan and heat until boiling. Add chicken and let simmer over medium heat, stirring frequently until chicken is cooked (it will turn completely white when cooked). Stir in onion and cook for 5 minutes. Add chiles and salsa and simmer for 10 minutes, stirring occasionally.

Spoon chicken mixture onto 2 cups of lettuce per serving, and top with tomato and scallions. Garnish with cheese and sour cream, if desired. Serve with Home-Style Tortilla Chips.

To make Home-Style Tortilla Chips, cook corn tortilla until crisp in microwave oven on high setting for 3 to 3½ minutes, turning once after 2 minutes, or in con-

ventional oven at 350 degrees for 7 to 8 minutes, turning once after 4 minutes; break into tortilla chips.
(Serves two)   ❧

Stuffed Baked Potato ❧

1 large russet potato

Stuffing Mixture (Delete if you binge on these foods):

1 ounce cheese, any low-fat type
1 tablespoon sautéed diced onions
1 tablespoon sautéed sliced mushrooms
½ cup cooked broccoli florets
¼ teaspoon salt-free seasoning blend (pepper, garlic,
onion combination)
1 tablespoon low-fat sour cream
1 tablespoon plain low-fat yogurt

Pierce skin of potato with fork and bake at 400 degrees
for 45 minutes, or on highest setting in microwave for
10 minutes. Cut potato in half lengthwise, scoop out
potato from skin. Set skins aside and put potato in
bowl. Mash potato; add 1 ounce cheese, sautéed (sliced
and cooked in margarine) onions and mushrooms,
cooked broccoli, seasoning blend, sour cream and yogurt. Whip mixture with fork or hand-held mixer on
low speed. Spoon mixture into potato skins and place
remaining cheese on top. Cook for 5 minutes at 400

degrees in conventional oven, or 1½ minutes on high in microwave. *(Serves one)* ❧

Chinese Stir-Fry ❧

1 teaspoon cooking oil
6 ounces chicken, skin and fat removed, shredded or sliced or lean beef (such as round steak), sliced into thin strips
1 large clove fresh garlic, pressed or diced★★
1 tablespoon soy sauce
½ brown onion, peeled and sliced into thin strips
½ green bell pepper, seeds removed, cut into thin slices
1 cup broccoli florets
5 scallions (green onions), diced
½ cup diced celery
1 cup large bean sprouts
5 large mushrooms, sliced

Heat cooking oil in non-stick skillet over medium-high heat until oil smokes slightly. Add chicken or beef and brown with garlic. Add soy sauce and stir until meat is completely cooked. Add all vegetables except bean sprouts and mushrooms, and stir continuously for 2 minutes. Then gently stir in bean sprouts and mushrooms, making sure vegetables and meat are completely mixed. Cook for 2 minutes. Serve with steamed white rice. *(Serves two)* ❧

Baked Cornish Game Hen with Wild Rice 🍃

1 cup wild rice
1 cup water
1 tablespoon low-calorie margarine
½ brown onion, peeled and diced
1 large clove garlic, pressed or diced★★
¼ teaspoon sage
¼ teaspoon parsley flakes
1 small cornish game hen, split in half

Preheat oven to 400 degrees. Put rice, water, margarine, onion, garlic, sage and parsley flakes in shallow glass pan and stir. Place game hen on top of rice mixture and put aluminum foil tent over pan. Bake for 1 hour, basting frequently with juice from the pan. Remove foil tent; brown for 15 minutes. *(Serves two)*   🍃

Eggplant Mozzarella 🍃

½ pound eggplant, cut into 4 to 6 thick slices
1 cup water

Italian Sauce

6 ounces tomato paste
1 teaspoon oregano★★
1 teaspoon marjoram
½ teaspoon thyme
¼ teaspoon sage
½ teaspoon salt
½ brown onion, peeled and diced
1 clove fresh garlic, pressed or diced★★
2 ounces mozzarella cheese, grated, or 4 tablespoons
low-fat cottage cheese if your binge food is cheese

Preheat oven to 450 degrees. Bake eggplant with ½ cup water in shallow glass pan for 10 minutes. While eggplant is baking, make Italian Sauce on stove top as follows: In medium-size pot, combine tomato paste, ½ cup water, spices, onion and garlic and mix well. Simmer for 20 minutes over medium heat, stirring often. Drain water from baking dish. Pour Italian Sauce over eggplant and cover with aluminum foil. Bake for 15 minutes. Remove foil and spread cheese or cottage cheese over mixture. Bake for 10 minutes, or until cheese is browned. *(Serves two)*

Baked Trout ❧

2 medium rainbow trout, deboned and butterflied
¼ cup water
½ teaspoon parsley flakes
½ teaspoon onion powder or flakes
¼ teaspoon garlic powder
1 teaspoon low-calorie margarine

Preheat oven to 425 degrees. Place trout in shallow glass pan with skin facing down and pour water and seasonings on top. Place ½ teaspoon margarine on each piece of trout. Bake uncovered for 15 minutes, basting frequently with juice from pan. *(Serves two)*   ❧

Sautéed Zucchini and Baby Carrots ❧

1 tablespoon low-calorie margarine
½ teaspoon onion powder
¼ teaspoon garlic powder
12 baby carrots, fresh or frozen
3 zucchini

Over medium heat, melt margarine in non-stick skillet and stir in spices. Place carrots in margarine mixture and stir frequently. Slice unpeeled zucchini and add to carrots. Cook until zucchini slices are slightly brown on each side. *(Serves two)*   ❧

Spanish-Style Chicken and Rice ❧

2 chicken breasts, skin and fat removed
2 tablespoons diced green chiles**
2 tablespoons salsa**
¼ brown onion, peeled and diced
⅔ cup uncooked white rice
1 cup grated monterey jack cheese or *1 cup cottage*
cheese if your binge food is cheese

Cook chicken (with bone in, if you like) in pot of boiling water until meat turns white. Run cold water over chicken to cool it off, then shred into small strips. In small frying pan, combine chicken, chiles, salsa, onion and 1 cup hot water. Simmer over low heat and stir frequently while steaming rice in a separate pot. Serve chicken mixture over rice and top with cheese or cottage cheese. *(Serves two)* ❧

Teriyaki Beef and Broccoli with Rice ❧

6 ounces lean steak (such as round)
3 tablespoons teriyaki sauce
1 cup water
2 cups broccoli florets
1 cup cooked white rice

Cut steak into strips approximately ½ inch wide by 3 inches long. In non-stick skillet, heat 1 tablespoon teriyaki sauce over medium-high heat. Add steak and stir constantly to brown meat. Then add broccoli and water and simmer until broccoli becomes slightly tender. Add rice and 2 tablespoons teriyaki sauce; stir until rice becomes light brown throughout and water is absorbed. *(Serves two)*   ❧

Barbecued Chicken Shish Kebabs ❧

3 chicken breasts, skin and fat removed
1 cup low-calorie italian salad dressing
1 green bell pepper
1 brown onion, peeled
12 cherry tomatoes
12 mushrooms

Cut chicken into approximately 1-inch cubes and soak in salad dressing for at least one hour. Cut bell pepper and onion into 1- to 2-inch chunks. Put marinated chicken and vegetables on separate shish kebab skewers. Cook chicken on barbecue grill before starting vegetables, turning chicken as needed. During the last 5 minutes of cooking time, put the vegetable skewers on the grill, and cook. *(Serves two)*   ❧

Sautéed Scallops 🍃

½ pound bay scallops
1 tablespoon low-calorie margarine
¼ brown onion, peeled and minced
½ cup white wine

Wash scallops and set aside. Slowly melt margarine in large skillet over low heat. Add minced onion and stir until onion becomes soft, clear and slightly brown on the edges. Add wine and increase heat to medium. Let mixture heat for approximately 3 minutes, stirring occasionally. Add scallops and stir while heating. Scallops are done when they turn completely white. *(Serves two)* 🍃

Cajun Snapper 🍃

1 pound red snapper fillets (2 large or 3 medium)
3 tablespoons water
½ tablespoon low-calorie margarine
1 tablespoon Cajun seasoning (marketed under various brand names in seasonings section of grocery stores)

Heat oven to 450 degrees. Put fillets in water in shallow glass pan. Divide margarine into two or three sections (depending on number of fillets you are preparing) and place 1 pat of margarine on each fillet. Sprinkle Cajun seasoning over top side of each fillet, making sure that seasoning is spread evenly and thinly and that it covers each fillet completely. When oven is hot, cook for 15 minutes. Check with fork to see if fish is flaky and done throughout; if not, cook for 5 more minutes. *(Serves two)* 🔊

9

Trimming and Toning Your Body

THROUGHOUT TIME, myriad diet clubs, books and dieting gurus have perpetuated myths and fantasies surrounding weight loss. One myth that unfortunately remains is that you can have a trimmed, toned and slim body without exercising.

I, like many dieters, fought the notion of mandatory exercise for a long time. I thought that I could beat the odds and be different—maybe other people needed to exercise, I'd rationalize, but not me. So I'd lose weight by vigorous dieting until my body was fairly slim. The trouble was, though, that it wasn't firm. My diet-thin body was still flabby, especially in my stomach, hips and thighs.

Dieting without exercise doesn't deliver the body of

your dreams! A dramatic example of this was seen in my patient Chris. Chris was 5 feet 4 inches tall and weighed 90 pounds. She was, as you may have guessed, suffering from anorexia nervosa. Chris had starved herself from her highest weight of 130 pounds to her present life-threatening weight. Because her weight was so low, and because Chris refused to eat enough to sustain her, she had to be hospitalized and fed intravenously.

While Chris was in the hospital, the staff took photographs of her while she was standing and clothed in her bra and panties. The purpose was to show Chris how she resembled a skeleton more than a slim fashion model. When she saw the photos of herself, Chris was shocked!

"I couldn't believe what I looked like!" Chris told me. "My hips and thighs were completely out of proportion with the rest of my body." It was true. Chris had believed she'd get the body of a high-fashion model if only she'd starve herself to a certain thinness. She never exercised, however—mostly because her starving made her too weak to do anything physical. But the striking thing for Chris was to realize that, without exercise, she'd never have the firm stomach and thighs that she dreamed of. Chris had starved herself into a cartoon-like, distorted version of her former self.

Today I have found, like Chris and many others, that exercise is a necessary component of maintaining a slim, healthy body. And the nice thing is that after two or three weeks of beginning an exercise program, you may start to look forward to exercising!

There are several other important benefits you'll get from exercise:

- Your weight loss will be faster.
- Your appetite will lessen, along with your cravings for binge foods and snacks.
- You will feel more energy during the day.
- You will sleep more soundly and awake more refreshed.
- You will find your stress level is reduced (great news for Stress Eaters!).
- You will find your fattening feelings are reduced (great news for Emotion Eaters!).

The exercise program described below is designed with the sedentary, non-motivated person in mind. I've tried to make a program that will *gradually* introduce you to a regular fitness routine. In this way, you'll be less apt to take one look at this chapter and say, "Oops! That's not for me."

Step #5 for Binge Eaters and Step #4 for All Other Yo-Yo Syndrome Sufferers: Develop Your Exercise Program

It's important to check with your physician before beginning any weight-loss or fitness program. This is especially true if you haven't had a checkup within the past six months or if you have a history of cardiovascular or muscular disorders.

The consensus among fitness experts is that aerobic activity—the kind that gets your heart pumping and your breathing really going—is the best way to lose fat, tone muscles and improve your cardiovascular fitness. Getting your heart rate up to target for at least 40 minutes at a time is generally considered better for your weight-loss program than exercising *less strenuously* for longer periods of time. That's why normal house work isn't a viable substitute for the type of aerobic exercise described below.

First, calculate what your target heart rate is by using the following formula:

Subtract your age from the number 220. The remainder is your "maximum heart rate"—the maximum number of beats per minute your heart should reach while you're exercising.

Next, multiply the remainder by .70 if you have been sedentary and not exercised for the past six months on a regular basis. If you're in good physical condition and regularly exercise, then multiply the remainder by .75. This figure is your "target heart rate," the number of beats per minute your heart should reach when you're exercising.

To calculate your heart rate while exercising, find your pulse with the tips of your index and middle fingers placed either on your neck or the inside of your wrist. With a stopwatch or the second hand on a regular watch, count your pulse for 6 seconds, then multiply this figure by 10. This is the number of beats per minute, or your current heart rate.

If your heart rate, at any time, exceeds your target heart rate, slow down the pace of your exercising (never stop suddenly, however). If your heart rate is 10 or more beats below your target heart rate, then speed up your pace or raise your arms above your head (this increases your heart rate).

CHOOSE YOUR EXERCISE PROGRAM

Ideally, you would choose one of the activities discussed below and perform it at your target heart rate for at least 40 continuous minutes four to five times a week. Don't exceed your target heart rate, as this will put you into the anaerobic process, in which you're no longer burning fat, but are instead building muscle. Always warm up slowly for at least 5 minutes before exercising aerobically, and cool down after exercising until your heart rate is at least 15 beats per minute below your target heart rate.

Low-Impact Aerobic Dance. This form of aerobics is different from traditional aerobics, where you bounce and swing your body in ways that make you prone to injury. Low-impact aerobic classes are offered at most gyms, on television programs and on video tape.

Jogging. Many people enjoy jogging before or after work. You may choose to jog around your neighborhood or on a track at a nearby school or college.

Rebounder (Trampoline) Jogging. This relatively inexpensive ($15 to $25) piece of exercise equipment is available at most department stores, and is ideal for people who prefer to exercise at home. There are at least two books out now that describe different ways to exercise on the rebounder. In addition, many people prefer to bounce holding five- to ten-pound weights or strapping weights on their wrists or ankles to increase the amount of calories they burn.

Swimming. You can burn calories and tone muscles by swimming laps back and forth across the pool or by doing calisthenics in the pool, letting the resistance of the water pump up your heart and calorie-burning rate.

Stair Climbing. This is my personal favorite. I use a StairMaster machine, which simulates walking, jogging or running up flights of stairs. Stair climbing is superb for toning the buttocks and legs (an area most women are concerned with), as well as burning calories and building cardiovascular fitness.

Most gyms have StairMaster machines these days. However, if yours doesn't, you can still get the benefit of stair climbing by stepping up and down on a small, sturdy box. Or you can imitate professional athletes by running up and down the grandstand steps at your local football field.

Bicycle Riding. If you don't own a bicycle, either stationary or conventional, think about investing in one. There's nothing more relaxing than pedaling to the

local grocery store or just tooling around the neighborhood at sunset.

Stationary bicycles are handy for at-home fitness
buffs, as you can park them in front of the television set
and pedal away as you watch your favorite show. I like
to exercise while watching the music video channel because the beautiful, slender models featured on most
videos inspire me to exercise and the beat of the music
motivates me.

Rowing. Rowing machines are another piece of
equipment that you can add to your home fitness center
or use at the local gym. Rowing is great for building up
a sweat and getting an aerobic workout, and it tones the
arms, chest and shoulders as well.

Tennis (or Racquetball). I like tennis because it's
necessarily a social sport, and exercising with a friend
can help keep Yo-Yo Syndrome Dieters motivated to
stick with their fitness programs. You and your tennis
partner can make sure you both get out on the court—
no excuses accepted.

Brisk Walking. This is another exercise that's best
done with a partner, either human or canine. Just don't
walk to the doughnut shop! (More walking information
below.)

Martial Arts. If you've ever felt physically vulnerable, unsure, or unsure you could protect yourself against
an attacker, why not take a karate or judo class? You'll

burn a lot of calories, get a good workout and feel safer. Most cities offer low-cost classes to the public—check your local yellow pages under "martial arts," or call your local parks and recreation department or community college.

The Walking Program

I realize that not everyone's going to gleefully jump into a fitness program. Many regard exercising as a chore, remembering grueling high school physical education classes when they had to run ten laps around the schoolyard. Some will say, "Well, I'll try the diet, but I'll just skip this exercise step." Others, who have been sedentary for six months or more, *shouldn't* start out right away with an aerobics program, but need instead to gradually incorporate exercise into their lifestyles.

Walking is a pain-free way to gradually introduce exercise into your life and help you burn some calories. Though this is not an aerobic program, it will start you in the right direction and perhaps inspire you to move on to an aerobic program later.

The walking program involves adding three activities to your normal daily routine:

1. Always park your car at the outer edge of the parking lot. This will give you the opportunity to walk to the store or work, and will also save your car from "parking lot dings."

2. Take the stairs instead of the elevator or escalator. You'll beat the crowds and will probably get to your destination faster than you would by waiting around for the elevator to arrive.

3. Once a day, go for a half-hour walk around the neighborhood. Make this a firm rule for yourself and always stick to it. After–dinner overeaters should get in the habit of getting out of the kitchen, out of the house, and outside into the fresh air. Homemakers, shift workers and those who work out of their homes should take morning walks to get their metabolism going and inspire them to stay away from temptation during the day. Exercise, once it is incorporated into your lifestyle, will have a ripple effect, creating a healthy mindset. After going to the time and trouble to exercise, you won't want to spoil your efforts with overeating.

If your schedule doesn't permit a walk because you get home so late at night (or if you don't feel safe walking around your neighborhood), go for a walk at the local shopping center or mall—just be sure to stay away from the bakery. Or walk in place while you watch your favorite television show.

What Kind of Exercise Do You Prefer?

Don't make the mistake of waiting until you're in the mood to begin an exercise program because that day may never come. Instead, push yourself to do something physical right now.

If you don't belong to a gym, then maybe it's time to join one. Exercising at home alone requires a tremendous amount of self-discipline, something most of us don't have when we're first starting a diet and fitness program. Pick a gym where you feel comfortable and that is located close enough to your home or work so that you'll actually go there at least four times a week.

Many Yo-Yo Syndrome sufferers are embarrassed to join a gym, thinking they're too fat to dance around in leotards or shorts in front of strangers. I understand this illogical logic, because I've thought the same thing in years past. It's kind of like wanting to clean your house before the maid arrives so she won't think you're a slob. However, don't fall into this trap now, because gyms are there to help you lose your excess weight. Besides, I've found that most people—male and female—working out at gyms are too absorbed in their own worlds to notice those exercising around them.

It's really important that you choose an activity that you enjoy, or it will be even more difficult to talk yourself into exercising. Think about your natural tendencies when deciding what type of exercise to engage in:

- Do you prefer to be alone? Then you'll probably do best exercising at home with a video tape or exercise equipment. Since you won't have anyone around urging you to exercise, you'll have to schedule exercise into your lifestyle. You may want to do this by pairing another activity that is already an ingrained habit—say, your 2 o'clock soap opera —with the exercise. This will trigger a reminder that it's time to watch "Days of Our Lives" *and* jog on the rebounder.

- Do you prefer to be with one other person? Then you may enjoy two-person sports such as tennis or racquetball. This may be an ideal situation, as well, if you and your exercise buddy make a pact to "bully" each other into working out on those days when you'd rather not.

- Do you like to be with a lot of other people? If so, then you'll probably like gyms, aerobics, martial arts or dance classes. At these places, you'll have the opportunity to introduce yourself to potential new friends.

- Do you like to be indoors? Then choose exercises that take place in gyms, racquetball courts, martial arts studios, dance halls, or indoor swimming pools, or exercise at home.

- Do you like to be outdoors? Then your sports would naturally be in league with tennis, bicycle riding, team sports, jogging or brisk walking.

There are other considerations to keep in mind as well, such as your budget. Some exercise plans, like racquetball or gym memberships, can run into a great deal of money by the time you finish paying for gym outfits, tennis shoes and club dues. Other programs, like brisk walking, cost practically nothing (although you should make sure to wear proper shoes no matter what exercise you choose).

Keep Yourself Motivated

How many times have you joined a gym, bought some home exercise equipment or committed yourself to a jogging regime, only to abandon it a month later? If you're like most Yo-Yo Syndrome sufferers, the answer's likely to be, "Too many times to remember."

Exercise, although such an important part of any weight-loss program, is usually the first thing to go when schedules get busy. For some, getting started is the hardest part. Once they get into a routine of exercising, they begin to enjoy it so much that they refuse to let it go. But for most of us, sticking with it is the hard part. We'll run, pump or swim ourselves into shape and then stop exercising for one reason or another. And when we stop working out, we often return to overeating.

This time, plan on sticking with your fitness routine! Just as for your diet, there are no stopping points for exercising. You don't just get in shape one day and say, "Okay, that's enough exercise. I'm done with it forever."

Here are some tips that will help you to stay with exercise. Try them out—they really do help!

- If you like the sport you've chosen, you're more likely to stick with it. Remember that it may take time to find the exercise that's right for you, so be patient if the one you're currently engaged in doesn't feel quite right. Instead of abandoning exercise entirely, switch to a different type.

- Schedule exercise into your day in the same way you would any important activity. Plan ahead which days and times would be best for you to exercise; note in pen on your calendar which days you plan to exercise. Try to be realistic in scheduling your exercise time to avoid setting yourself up for frustrations. Also, plan your exercise around your peak energy time (for example, if you're a "morning person," plan to exercise in the morning), and you'll feel more up to working out.

- Don't look at exercise as optional. Just as you wouldn't dream of missing that important meeting or doctor's appointment, keep your promise to yourself and exercise every time it's written on your calendar.

- If you begin to argue with yourself about why you don't have time to exercise, *stop!* Don't give yourself time to even think about it. You don't stop and argue with yourself about whether to take a shower every day, do you? Of course not! Do you stop and say, "Well, I don't have time to brush my hair and my teeth"? No. Put exercise into this category of things you "of course" do, just like showering and dressing.

- Buy a new exercise outfit or some new tennis shoes. There's nothing like feeling attractive to give you incentive to exercise. Just as you feel more excited about going to work when dressed in a flattering new outfit, you'll feel more charged about exercising if you know you look your best.

- Reward yourself for exercising, but wait until after

your workout to give yourself the reward. For instance, you can withhold your evening snack until after you're done working out. Or put a dollar into a piggy bank every time you exercise and spend it on yourself once a week or month.

- Team sports can add fun to your exercise program as well as keep you motivated (there's nothing like a play-off schedule to force you to exercise). Call your local parks and recreation department or community college and ask about joining their volleyball, soccer or softball teams.

- Consider hiring a personal trainer. This person will help you construct a fitness routine to suit your goals and needs. Then the trainer will stand with you during your entire workout—either at your home or the gym—to make sure you complete each exercise safely and thoroughly. To find out the cost of a trainer (some even work on the barter system—just ask them), call your local gyms.

- Exercising with a friend is another way to keep your motivation high, have fun and have someone to talk to while you work out. Make a pact with one another to not accept any excuses about not exercising, and you'll be able to push each other into sticking with a fitness routine.

- Like dieting, take your exercise progress one day at a time. Set small goals for yourself and have patience as you gradually increase your running distance, build aerobic stamina or lift progressively more weight. Try not to compare yourself to others, except as a way to set future goals for yourself.

- No excuses (except illness or injury) are acceptable for missing your exercise. If, after being brutally honest with yourself about your reasons, you decide you really can't exercise this morning as you planned, then reschedule your workout for this evening. Remember, excuses won't get the weight off of you!

- Some people drop out of exercise programs because they've overdone it and experienced "exercise burnout." Be realistic when scheduling exercise into your life, and keep a balance between too little and too much of a workout.

- Going away to a hotel for the weekend or for a business conference? Don't let your fitness routine be interrupted (this often breaks the pattern of exercising, and may cause you to stop your fitness program altogether). Make your reservations only at hotels that feature workout rooms, gyms, or jogging paths.

- I, as well as many of my clients, have found that aerobic exercise sparks creative ideas. For that reason, you might want to carry a small tape recorder or paper and pencil as you work out to capture your ideas as they occur. This benefit will help reinforce the rewards of exercising, especially for Stress Eaters who often claim they have too much work to do to stop to exercise.

- Finally, if your motivation to exercise is *really* low, try my 15-Minute Personal Pact. Tell yourself, "I'll exercise for 15 minutes. If, after 15 minutes, I feel like stopping, I will stop. After all, 15 minutes of exercise is better than nothing." I can virtually guarantee you that after 15 minutes, you'll want to keep going and you'll end up exercising for your 40-minute workout!

This step, to exercise regularly, is as important as any of the other steps in the Yo-Yo Syndrome Diet, so don't try to work around it. Too many studies confirm that toned, trim bodies are the result of combining a low-calorie, low-fat diet with exercise. Remember, exercise is not optional!

10

Restaurants and Your Eating Plan

Y O-YO Syndrome sufferers often worry how to stay on the Diet while away from home. Because of the myriad pressures and temptations that arise when you go "out there," Yo-Yo Syndrome sufferers do need to stay on guard to avoid overeating and subsequent weight gains.

Although I have one client who actually tried to arrange her life so that she never had to eat a meal away from home, most of us can't—or don't want to—avoid eating in restaurants, friends' houses or parties. And you don't have to on this eating plan, because it's designed to allow you to eat as close to "normal" as possible.

This chapter will give you some tools for survival

and some ways to keep your Yo-Yo Syndrome in check. But by far the greatest tool that you'll carry with you, both in your home and out, is the knowledge that you alone are responsible for what goes in your mouth (or on your thighs or belt line!). No matter what pressures come up in your life, no matter how guilty you may feel about saying "no" to someone's cooking, remember that you are in control of what enters your mouth.

Eating Out and Eating Thin

When dining out, you'll have to be very honest with yourself about how much food you're going to eat. Restaurants are notorious for serving extra-big portions of food—usually the equivalent of two servings appears on the large plate set before you. Since the Yo-Yo Syndrome Diet entails eating only one serving of whatever you eat, you'll need to stop eating when you start to feel full. Use your honest judgment and the guidelines in Chapters 7 and 8 to figure out how much food equals one serving. But, yes, I realize that the temptation to eat the whole thing often wins out, so here are some tips that may help:

- Before ordering, look at the size of the meals being served to the other restaurant patrons. Do they look like normal, medium or giant-sized portions?
- If they look gigantic, ask your waiter if you can

order a half-meal. Most restaurants are more than happy to accommodate such requests. And by having a smaller meal in front of you, you'll be less tempted to overeat.

- If you feel comfortable with the idea, why not split a gigantic meal with your dining companion? Even if there's a slight extra charge for splitting a meal, it's worth it.

- Remember that leaving food on your plate isn't wasteful. What is wasteful is eating more than you need and being angry at yourself for the extra weight you may subsequently gain.

- As soon as you begin to feel full (not stuffed), do one of the following before you even have time to think about eating more: throw your napkin over the plate so you won't see the rest of the food on the plate; or take someone's cigarette and put it out in the food to make it unappetizing to you; or sprinkle pepper all over the food on your plate, again to take away its appeal.

Don't even let yourself entertain the notion of eating more food if you're full. Push your plate to the edge of the table so that it'll be taken away. After 10 or 15 minutes, your brain should catch up with your stomach and register signals that it's full of food. In the meantime, you can go to the restroom and brush your teeth (be sure to carry a toothbrush and toothpaste with you wherever you go). Then order a cup of coffee so you won't feel empty-handed if your dining companions are still eating.

"Waiter, There's a Binge Food in My Soup!" —A Word to Binge Eaters

If you're a Binge Eater, don't play the game that so many do (I used to play this one myself): you see that the food on your plate or the food being offered to you contains your binge food. It looks delicious. You want it. So you tell yourself, "I can pretend I didn't know my binge food was in this and then it really wouldn't be my fault if I ate it." Yeah, it may not be your "fault" that you ate the food, but you'll be the one left on an eating binge. You'll be the one who feels fat, miserable and out of control. That's why it's vital to take responsibility for your diet.

If you ever come up against that panic-stricken dilemma of trying to decide, "Should I eat my binge food, or shouldn't I?", remember that you really don't even have the option. If you eat the binge food, you will end up relapsing—either today or in the next few days. And binges are not to be taken lightly, because they're difficult to stop and damaging to the self-esteem.

Remember: "If it is to be, it's up to me."

Going to a restaurant doesn't mean a struggle with your binge food—there are plenty of ways to stay on your Yo-Yo Syndrome Diet and feel very satisfied with your meal. I know, because I eat a lot of meals in restaurants and I've never had to forsake eating to stay on my diet (although I *would* go without eating before I'd eat my binge food).

The main thing to keep in mind when you eat out is

that even a little taste of your binge food can trigger
overeating, so carefully investigate how the meal is prepared before you order it. Don't be shy about asking
waiters and waitresses questions about the dish; they
expect to provide information as a part of the service
you're paying for.

Bread bingers should always ask if meat dishes are
breaded, or if the soup is made with flour. Ask that the
side of toast, biscuits or bread either not be served, be
served to your non-bread-binging eating companion or
be replaced by an extra portion of vegetables.

Sugar bingers should ask whether sugar is included
in the ingredients of the meal, especially if it's hidden in
sources such as sauces for meats, vegetables and salads.

Salty junk food bingers need to especially avoid deep-
fried, crunchy foods and so should take care to ask how
meat dishes are prepared.

Spicy food bingers should ask whether ingredients
can be substituted to tone down the intensity of the
meal. These days, the better restaurants are accustomed
to preparing low-sodium menus and special requests are
welcomed. Feel free to ask for meals low in all spices,
and you should find that your request is accommodated
with grace. If not, maybe you shouldn't eat in that restaurant anymore. Or you can stick with the so-called
American dishes, usually listed in the back of menus at
most ethnic restaurants, meals that are virtually guaranteed to be blander than ethnic dishes.

Dairy product bingers need to find out if their binge
food is involved in the meal's preparation. If your binge
food is cheese, then ask to have the order prepared with-

out it—a very reasonable request that shouldn't give
you any trouble from the restaurant staff. Make sure,
before you order, that your meal won't be smothered
with white sauce. And, of course, order a non-dairy
dressing with your dinner salad.

Each type of restaurant offers a different set of foods
that potentially contain your binge food as an ingredient, so I've listed the most common below. Most importantly, I've written some suggestions for what foods
you'd probably do best with and enjoy the most. A lot
of what follows tells you what foods to avoid rather
than what to have. As long as you avoid your binge
food, you should be able to eat happily and heartily no
matter where you are.

The Restaurant Survival Guide

The pages that follow outline which foods in different
types of restaurants fit into the Yo-Yo Syndrome Diet.
The foods are broken down into Binge Food categories—Yo-Yo Syndrome sufferers who are not Binge
Eaters should follow the guidelines for Sugar Bingers
and Salty Junk Food Bingers since these categories contain foods dieters must limit to keep their calorie count
down.

Remember, when you're dining out, to use the
guidelines for the Diet (as outlined in Chapters 7 and 8)
to help you decide what to order.

By using the descriptions below, you should be able

to stay on your Yo-Yo Syndrome Diet in any type of restaurant. However, if you're in doubt, be sure to ask your waiter or waitress for help. Tell him or her that you'd like a meal, for example, consisting of chicken, rice and vegetables, and your server should be able to suggest a meal on the menu that will fit the bill for you.

SALAD AND SOUP BARS

There was a time when I thought anything coming under the heading of "salad" was automatically low-calorie and good for me. It was a combination diet and health food, right? Well, fortunately most of us have caught on that all salads aren't necessarily created equal, and we're savvy to the fact that a mile-high pile of greens and beans topped with blue cheese dressing can easily tower to the 1200-calorie mark.

And while the Yo-Yo Syndrome Diet is not about counting calories, we don't want to completely disregard them either. Nor should we ignore fat, which has calories that turn into body fat four times faster than the same number of calories from another source.

Another general rule for dealing with salad and soup bars is to keep in mind that these "all-you-can-eat" situations are ripe for creating binges. To avoid overeating, remember to have only one serving of whatever you choose to eat. You might also limit the *number* of items you put on your salad; for instance, allowing yourself a maximum of six salad bar items will encourage moderation.

Bread Bingers

Avoid croutons, chips and breadsticks, of course. And when choosing a soup, stay away from the creamy or stew varieties as they are almost always thickened with flour (if in doubt, ask the restaurant staff). Instead of having clam chowder, cream of broccoli, or beef stew, have a bowl of chicken vegetable soup. Be sure to avoid soups containing noodles of any type.

Watch out for noodles and pasta, which are often hidden in salads. I've found that some noodles, when mixed in salads, often look like bean sprouts, so be sure to look at salads carefully before spooning those exotic mixtures onto your plate. You can test for noodles by fishing the suspect out of the salad with your fork and then cutting it with your silverware. A noodle will cut easily; a bean sprout will be crisper and resist cutting.

Bread bingers must stay alert for their particular variety of bread binge foods. For example, most bread bingers have to abstain from all forms of wheat and flour. Others can't tolerate any grains without going on a binge and so they must also abstain from rye, rice and barley.

Sugar Bingers

You've got quite a few things to avoid at the salad bar, believe it or not. This includes the so-called salads that are actually more in the dessert category, like gelatin, carrot salad, fruit salad made with whipped cream, canned fruits in sugary syrup and mousse.

It's also important to stay away from salad dressings containing sugar, such as french, russian or thousand island. Your best bet is to use a white salad dressing such as ranch style or blue cheese or the low-calorie dressing that most salad bars offer, or to mix oil and vinegar yourself. Be sure to avoid raisins, dates, banana chips and shredded coconut as well, as these all contain high amounts of natural and processed sugar. Most soups available don't contain sugar, so you really won't have to worry about that part of your meal.

Salty Junk Food Bingers

Like the bread binger, you should stay away from the fried or crunchy salad toppings, such as croutons, breadsticks, potato skins, tortilla chips and potato chips. In addition, avoid the following like the plague: nuts, crispy chinese noodles and bacon bits. Some of these binge foods are hidden in the salad mixtures, so be careful. For instance, many fruit salads are heavily laden with walnuts, and you could find yourself wanting to binge after a helping of this. Be kind to yourself and stay away from all the little, salty, crispy foods—most of the brown things—at the salad bar. Similarly, when eating soup, don't eat crackers of any kind.

Spicy Food Bingers

Your task, of course, is to avoid the intensely spicy foods that may lead to a binge. At a salad bar, this means avoiding the tangy or peppery mixtures such as pasta salad, salsa and marinated vegetables. Instead, choose the creamy mixtures such as fish salad and fruit salad, as they're usually tasty without being too bland. Use your eyes to look for signs of spiciness in foods— you can see peppers and onions most of the time. Top your salad with a mild dressing, such as french or thousand island. Spicy food bingers should be able to eat most soups, since they tend to be low-key in their flavor, but be very honest with yourself about what foods would trigger a binge in you.

Dairy Food Bingers

You'll have a few things to avoid at the salad and soup bar, too, although you're lucky because your binge food is harder to hide in the array of foods before you. Stay away from shredded cheese, blue cheese dressings, ranch-style dressings, whipped cream and sour cream, of course. And avoid any white, creamy salads since they may contain a dairy product that could spell doom for your recovery program.

As far as soups go, the rules are the same: steer clear of creamy, milky soups like chowders, cheese soups and cream of vegetable, and choose instead a clear brothy soup like chicken noodle or beef stew.

CHINESE RESTAURANTS

Chinese food has always been a favorite among dieters because of its high use of vegetables and other low-calorie ingredients. My only complaint about Chinese restaurants is their tendency to use monosodium glutamate (MSG) much too liberally. This salty flavor-enhancer makes almost everyone retain *a lot* of water for a day or two after eating it, so get in the habit of asking to have your food prepared without MSG. Almost every Chinese restaurant I've frequented is more than glad to offer this choice, as more and more people are opting to delete MSG from their diets.

Bread Bingers

Here are the foods for you to avoid at Chinese restaurants: anything that's made with tempura (a flour batter), egg rolls, wontons, crispy or soft noodles, moo-shu (Chinese-style pancakes), sweet-and-sour foods (they usually contain battered and fried pieces of meat and the sauce is thickened with flour), fortune cookies, and almond cookies.

You can enjoy any of the meals that are made of meat, fish and vegetables.

Sugar Bingers

For you, the Chinese restaurant won't pose much of a threat to your Yo-Yo Syndrome Recovery Program, with just a few things to watch out for. The only foods containing sugar in most Chinese restaurants are sweet-and-sour dishes, some sauces used to prepare duck, some dips offered with egg rolls, barbecue sauce on spareribs, and both fortune and almond cookies. Other than these, you can feel confident about ordering anything on the menu and safely avoiding your binge foods.

Salty Junk Food Bingers

You'll want to stay away from the Chinese equivalent of potato chips: crispy fried noodles. There's also a flake-type chip served in some restaurants that reminds me of corn flakes or unsweetened frosted flakes; stay away from this, as well. In addition, be sure to avoid the meals that are prepared with nuts, such as almond chicken, cashew chicken and kun pao chicken (which contains peanuts). Since most Chinese restaurants seem to be extremely generous in adding nuts to these dishes, I wouldn't attempt to order these meals under the assumption that you could avoid the almonds, cashews or peanuts—don't even tempt yourself!

Egg rolls and tempura, which are deep-fried, may trigger binges with some salty junk food bingers, so use utmost honesty with yourself if you think you compulsively overeat these Chinese foods. All in all, you'd be best to stick to the "soft" dishes, containing noodles and meat.

Spicy Food Bingers

Since most Chinese food is of an evenly low-key flavor and intensity, you aren't likely to binge. The exception, of course, is Szechuan cuisine, which you should steer completely away from. The menu should clearly differentiate the Szechuan meals from the others, but if you're in doubt, be sure to ask your waiter or waitress which dishes are hot and spicy.

Some spicy food bingers have trouble with some borderline spicy Chinese foods, so pay attention to your reaction to these. If you find yourself wanting to binge, then put these on your abstinence list: barbecued spareribs, barbecued chicken, sweet-and-sour dishes and beef with scallions (green onions).

Dairy Food Bingers

I have yet to see any dairy products offered in Chinese restaurants, with the exception of a white salad dressing one place offers, and of course ice cream. Other than these, you won't find a shred of cheese or a dollop of sour cream in a Chinese establishment, so relax and enjoy your meal without worry!

ITALIAN RESTAURANTS AND PIZZA PARLORS

Most dieters view pasta and pizza as no-no food. So Italian restaurants and pizza parlors are typically shunned by calorie-conscious Yo-Yo Syndrome sufferers. But this doesn't have to be. Many Italian dishes, and yes, even pizza, fit into the Yo-Yo Syndrome Diet as long as you follow your eating plan to control portions of meat, bread, dairy products and vegetables.

A word of caution, though, for all Yo-Yo Syndrome sufferers: many of the meats in Italian food are high in fat and sodium, so avoid pepperoni, salami, sausage of any type, mortadella and bacon. Instead, stick to meat dishes lower in fat, such as poultry and seafood, and choose low-fat pizza toppings like mushrooms, pineapple, bell peppers or jalapeño peppers. Olives, a traditional pizza topping, are also somewhat high in fat (4 grams of fat in just two black olives!), so limit or avoid eating them, as well.

Bread Bingers

Many bread bingers, when they go on the Yo-Yo Syndrome Diet, assume that they'll never again be able to eat at an Italian restaurant. "What would I eat?" they ask me incredulously. Well, let's briefly review first what *not* to eat: pasta such as lasagna and spaghetti, noodles such as fettucine and bread such as pizza crust, breadsticks and sandwich bread.

"Isn't that *everything* in an Italian restaurant?"

No, because as a bread binger myself, I'm able to walk into any Italian restaurant or pizza parlor and enjoy a delicious, satisfying and abstinent meal. And you can too. The first rule is "caveat emptor"—let the buyer beware. This means asking lots of questions about the preparation of the meals you want to order. In general, you can eat the following *unless* you find out that it has been breaded or contains noodles before being cooked (if it has, then ask to have it prepared without bread and/or noodles): chicken cacciatore, a side of meatballs, eggplant, veal or chicken parmigiana, antipasto salad, and any entrée in the same general category of unbreaded meat covered with spaghetti sauce and/or cheese. In addition, you can enjoy the top of a pizza. In other words, pull the cheese, meat and sauce away from the pizza crust and I think you'll find it very enjoyable.

Sugar Bingers

Sugar bingers have to beware of one thing in Italian restaurants and pizza parlors: sugar is often hidden in the spaghetti and pizza sauce. In better, family-style restaurants, the sauce is made without sugar. Don't discount this as a trivial point, because hidden sources of binge foods lead to compulsive overeating episodes in the same way that obvious sources do. Be sure to ask your waiter or waitress to find out if the sauces have sugar in them. And don't just take this person's guess about it, either. Ask him or her to check with the cook to see if sugar is one of the ingredients. If it is, ask if special arrangements can be made so that your sauce is made without sugar (it's okay to request special service —you're worth it, and besides, you're paying for it!). If this isn't possible, then have a dish without spaghetti sauce, such as pasta with clam, pescatore or calamari sauce.

And, of course, spumoni and other Italian desserts trigger binges, too.

Salty Junk Food Bingers

For you, the same guidelines apply here as in other restaurants. In general, watch out for the crunchy and fried foods. This means breadsticks, salad croutons, crunchy pizza crust (such as crunchy style or the edges of the pizza), and fried sandwiches.

The salty junk food binger will do best to stick with softer foods, such as noodle and meat dishes. If you do order pizza, be sure to order a soft-crust style and don't eat the edges.

Spicy Food Bingers

You may want to think long and hard before going to an Italian restaurant or pizza parlor, because it's difficult to avoid spicy foods in these places. In fact, it's kind of a cruel joke to play on yourself to even go into one—almost like a recovering alcoholic going into a bar.

However, if you do go into an Italian restaurant or pizza parlor, your best bet would probably be to eat an antipasto or chef's salad, or a milder pasta dish such as noodles with white sauce. Stay away from anything red, such as pepperoni, spaghetti sauce and pizza.

Dairy Food Bingers

Like the spicy food binger, you may want to avoid Italian restaurants and pizza parlors because of the abundance of cheese used in these places. About the only dish offered without cheese would be a plate of spaghetti (hold the parmesan, please!) or cheeseless chicken cacciatore.

Again, don't be shy about asking for help from your waiter or waitress in dealing with your Yo-Yo Syndrome. Explain to the person that you have an allergy to dairy products (you do, after all!) and would he or she please help you order a meal that has no cheese in it. The restaurant employee should be more than happy to help you—if not, I wouldn't return to that place and I'd be sure to tell the manager about it, as well.

MEXICAN RESTAURANTS

The two Mexican food ingredients that all Yo-Yo Syndrome sufferers should avoid are refried beans with lard and guacamole. These side dishes and ingredients in many foods are much too high in fat to be in anyone's diet. Ask to have your meal prepared without them.

Bread Bingers

Foods to avoid include tortillas and tortilla products, such as tortilla chips (push that basket of chips far, far away from you!), taco shells, tostada shells, taquitos, enchilada tortillas and burrito tortillas. In addition, you'll need to stay away from breaded foods such as chile rellenos. Nevertheless, there are lots of great foods at Mexican restaurants you'll probably enjoy.

Your best bets are foods based on meat and vegetables. You also can eat the insides (lettuce, cheese, meat, etc.) of tostadas and tacos—just be careful to not eat any of the shell.

Sugar Bingers

To my knowledge, all Mexican dishes are prepared without sugar, with the exception of desserts, pastries and sweet breads. However, I'd be sure to ask if you have any doubts about the ingredients of a dish, including anything that has a sweet sauce poured on it. And, of course, margaritas are loaded with sugar!

Salty Junk Food Bingers

You'll need to beware of crunchy taco chips and tortillas, as well as *crisp* fried foods such as deep-fried burritos. That means avoiding crispy tacos, tostada shells and taquitos. Look instead for *soft* foods such as burritos (made without refried beans), *soft* tacos or meat-and-vegetable dishes.

Spicy Food Bingers

As with Italian food, spicy food bingers are entering a den of binge foods when they walk into a Mexican restaurant. For that reason, why not be kind to yourself and eat elsewhere instead? However, if you find yourself in a Mexican restaurant (at, say, a company dinner), then be sure to order an "American" dish. This type of meal usually consists of a steak, broiled without salsa. Have a green salad as your side dish, and avoid spanish rice or anything else that's spicy, hot or potentially binge-triggering.

Dairy Food Bingers

Most Mexican food is topped with cheese and sour cream, but you'll still be able to eat at this type of restaurant by avoiding these two dairy products. I've had many clients who learned to enjoy tacos without cheese and sour cream, but if this doesn't sound appealing to you, order meals that don't normally come with these toppings. Foods such as camarones (broiled shrimp) or fajitas taste great in such a way that cheese or sour cream won't be missed.

AMERICAN RESTAURANTS

Whether it's a roadside stand, a 24-hour diner, a nationally known franchise or an exquisite restaurant with valet parking, American food usually signifies steak, roast beef, ham, chicken, seafood and such. These meals are simple but filling, moderate in temperature and spices, and almost everyone enjoys them.

Bread Bingers

It's fitting to start this discussion with the first meal of the day, since most American restaurants serve breakfast. Of course, your abstinence from bread means avoiding pancakes, waffles, crêpes (they're made with flour), biscuits and muffins. It's also a good idea to avoid hash browns, unless you're absolutely certain you don't binge on this starchy (and oily!) dish. Instead, your breakfast could consist of eggs, an omelette, yogurt, or fresh fruit with cottage cheese.

For lunch and dinner, foods to avoid are sandwich breads (although you *can* eat the meat, cheese, and lettuce of the sandwich without the bread), hamburger or hot dog buns (again, feel free to eat the meat without the bread), french fries, onion rings, breaded meats, flour-based creamy soups, flour-based gravy, noodles, pasta, salad croutons and crackers.

Instead, dine on chef's salad, fruit with cottage cheese or any meat-with-vegetable combination. You can enjoy any unbreaded chicken, beef, pork or fish plate with vegetables and rice (unless rice is a binge food for you). Give the complimentary biscuit or bread to your dining companion, or ask if you can substitute something "edible" such as an extra helping of vegetables for the bread.

Sugar Bingers

Sugar bingers will need to watch out for hidden sources of sugar, so they should have the same sort of breakfast as bread bingers. Sugar is often an ingredient in the batter used to make pancakes, waffles, nut or banana bread, muffins and crêpes, so even if you were to eat these foods *without* syrup, you'd still be eating sugar. The only baked goods you can count on to not have sugar are biscuits and plain bread or toast.

For some reason, many American restaurants serve canned fruit with sugary syrup instead of fresh fruit. Sugar bingers should exercise extreme caution before eating fruit at a restaurant, because the syrup can trigger a binge. Along the same lines, I've had a few sugar binger clients who found that the new "sugarless" jellies (those sweetened only with fruit juice) also triggered eating binges in them. It seems that the concentrated fruit sugars in these jellies—like the ones in raisins or dates—set off an eating binge in the same way that processed sugar does. Be cautious with all these forms of sugar when ordering from the menu. In addition, most commercial brands of cereal contain sugar; the ones that don't usually brag about it, printing big announcements such as "No Sugar Added" across the front of the package. However, restaurants rarely carry the sugarless brands of cereal.

Your best bet for breakfast is to have any of the following: eggs, an omelette, bacon, ham, hash browns, toast, biscuits or fresh fruit with cottage cheese.

Lunch and dinner foods can also contain hidden sugars. Watch out for such foods as apple rings, salad dressings (almost all, even the low-calorie varieties, are made with sugar—with the exception of make-it-yourself oil and vinegar dressings), sweet sauces such as barbecue or ketchup, sweet pickles, tuna salad, candied yams or carrots, and applesauce.

Sugar bingers do have a large selection to choose from for these two meals, however, since most American lunches and dinners consist of meat and vegetables. You'll be safe if you eat something like shrimp, chicken, hamburgers (avoid sauce containing sugar, however), turkey, ham, steak, pasta, fish, roast beef, salads with blue cheese or italian dressing, vegetables, soups, rice, or potatoes.

Salty Junk Food Bingers

Once again, the salty junk food binger's task is to avoid the crunchy, fried types of food which, unfortunately, are the hallmark of American restaurants. For breakfast, you'll be on the safe side as long as you avoid fried foods such as hash browns, french toast and crêpes. Some salty junk food bingers find that they binge on crispy bacon, so if this causes you to overeat you'll want to avoid it.

Lunch and dinner follow the same guidelines, so you're free to have anything on the menu except fried, crispy foods such as fried sandwiches (like grilled cheese), cheese or garlic bread, onion rings, potato chips, pretzels, nuts, french fries, and fried meats.

Enjoy a meal, if you like, consisting of non-fried foods such as roasted chicken, turkey with gravy, grilled steak, hamburger, ham, broiled (not fried) fish or roast beef. For side dishes, you could have rice (although watch out for pilafs and vegetable dishes containing nuts), vegetables, mashed or baked potatoes, salad (no croutons, though), soup, fruit or applesauce.

Spicy Food Bingers

You should be able to find plenty of food in an American restaurant that won't trigger a binge for you. Since most American food is made with moderate amounts of spices, you'll probably be able to order anything on the menu without any worry at all.

For breakfast, meals to avoid would be omelettes containing onions, bell peppers, chili or salsa; spicy sausage, and hash browns made with onions. Choose instead foods like pancakes, waffles, muffins, bacon, ham, cereal, eggs or fruit with cottage cheese.

Lunch and dinner foods to stay away from would include anything "ethnic" on the menu (e.g., Mexican, Cajun, Italian, etc.), spicy sauces such as barbecue or horseradish (which is also an ingredient in shrimp sauce), garlic bread, chili, spicy versions of baked beans or onions. Anything *but* these spicy foods and condiments would be perfect for the spicy food binger.

Dairy Food Bingers

For breakfast, the dairy food binger must take into consideration what his or her particular binge foods are. As mentioned before, some dairy food bingers binge on *just* one or two specific types of dairy products (such as cheese, ranch-style dressing, sour cream or frozen yogurt). They are able to eat virtually any other type of dairy food and don't feel tempted, in the least, to overeat.

This is where the Yo-Yo Syndrome Diet again differs from conventional diets: only you, by being rigorously honest with yourself, know which foods you can and cannot eat. So this discussion will look at *all* the dairy products offered at American restaurants. If you binge on all dairy foods, then you'll need to abstain from all of them. If, on the other hand, you binge only on one or two of them, then by all means avoid those particular foods.

Breakfast dairy products are found in quite a few of the meals on the menu. Eggs, cheese, butter, cottage cheese, milk, sour cream and whipped cream are ingredients in such dishes as pancakes, waffles, crêpes, muffins and biscuits. If you need to abstain from all dairy products, then you'll be sticking to a meal of meat (bacon, ham), hash browns and/or fruit. Since meats and fried hash browns are so high in fat and cholesterol, I wouldn't recommend eating them more than once or twice a week. Instead, eat plenty of fresh fruit.

For lunch and dinner, you'll be faced with fewer dairy products on the menu, but there still are plenty of meals containing cheese, white sauces and gravies, sour cream, dairy-based salad dressings (ranch-style, thousand island, french and blue cheese) and white soups. In addition, anything with bread (e.g., fried foods, baked goods, sandwiches) has dairy products in it.

This means the Yo-Yo Syndrome sufferer who

binges on all dairy products should eat meals consisting of unbreaded meats with no white sauces or cheese on them, vegetables with seasoned salt instead of butter, unbuttered rice, potatoes seasoned with chives or salt instead of butter or sour cream, salad with italian or russian dressing, and fruit.

FAST-FOOD RESTAURANTS

If I had written this section ten years ago, my task would have been simple because fast-food fare at that time consisted solely of hamburgers and french fries. Today, there are so many different foods available in fast-food restaurants that I couldn't possibly describe them all here. Even as this book is being published, there are certain to be new varieties of fast food available to the public. This discussion, therefore, will largely apply to the traditional "hamburger joints" such as McDonald's and Burger King.

Yes, you can eat at a fast-food restaurant! The Yo-Yo Syndrome Diet really does allow you to eat anywhere. I would caution you against consuming a whole lot of fatty red meats, however, because the calories in fat turn into body fat so quickly. While it's still possible to lose weight and eat hamburgers, your weight loss will be much quicker if you limit your fat intake to roughly 20 percent of your total daily food intake. An easy way to cut the amount of fat in your diet is to avoid eating red meats (beef and pork), fried foods and whole milk products as much as possible, or at least keep your intake of them to a maximum of once a week.

Bread Bingers

For you, the key to eating at fast-food restaurants is to avoid buns of any kind. This means if you want a hamburger or hot dog, you need to eat the meat, sauce and lettuce without the bun. I've done this for years and have learned to prefer my fast food this way. You can either order the hamburger and hot dog, and then throw away the bun yourself, or you can order what is called a "K-9" version of the meal. That means a hamburger or hot dog without the bun, named such because dog owners sometimes order bun-less hamburgers and hot dogs for their pets when going through a drive-through. Other bread products to avoid include sandwich breads, pita bread and biscuits.

In addition, you'll need to avoid the breaded side dishes offered at some places, such as fried zucchini, chicken nuggets or mushrooms. As mentioned before, many bread bingers also can't tolerate fried potatoes such as french fries or chips, so these should be avoided as well.

I'm so happy to see fast-food restaurants offering salads these days. Bread bingers can enjoy salads as long as they avoid croutons. Another item that many bread bingers may be able to eat (depending on the individual) is a stuffed potato—that is, a baked potato filled with butter, sour cream, broccoli or bacon. Keep in mind, however, that these ingredients—except broccoli, of course—are full of fat and need to be eaten in moderation.

Sugar Bingers

With the exception of hamburger sauce (the thousand island type), shakes, salad dressings, barbecue sauce, hot dog relish, desserts and non-diet sodas, sugar bingers will find plenty of safe foods in a fast-food restaurant.

You can eat hamburgers, cheeseburgers or hot dogs, as long as you stay away from the sugary condiments (for instance, order your hamburger without sauce and avoid ketchup, as it contains lots of sugar—have mustard, mayonnaise or seasoned salt instead). You can also enjoy salad with oil and vinegar, chicken nuggets (with an unsugared sauce) or a stuffed potato.

Salty Junk Food Bingers

Your best bet would be to stay away from all fast-food restaurants!

Seriously, most of the foods in these establishments are fried or crispy, so you'll probably be tempted like crazy. However, if you do go into a fast-food place (say you're on a road trip and there's nothing else around), be sure to avoid the following: french fries, onion rings, potato chips, fried hamburgers (eat only grilled or charbroiled), popcorn, chicken nuggets, crunchy salad toppings, fried vegetables and grilled breads.

Instead, stick with the softer foods available at the restaurant, such as a sandwich, hot dog, stuffed potato (without bacon), charbroiled hamburger or salad. And

be sure to hold yourself to the Yo-Yo Syndrome Diet
guideline of one serving only, because the smells of
french fries and hamburgers in a fast-food restaurant
often make salty junk food bingers have cravings.

Spicy Food Bingers

You shouldn't have much trouble finding non-binge
foods at fast-food restaurants, because like American
restaurants, they offer food that for the most part is
pretty mild or bland. Feel free to order anything on the
menu, but ask the cook to hold the onions on your
hamburger (or grill them, which reduces their spiciness)
and refrain from adding extra salt and pepper to your
burger.

There are also some fast-food restaurants that
smother their hamburgers and fries with chili—a meal
you'll need to avoid, of course. Other establishments
put heavy amounts of seasoned or onion salt on their
french fries, a practice that could lead to a binge for
you. Therefore, ask how the french fries are prepared if
you have any doubts. Some spicy food bingers overeat
onion rings; if you do, too, then be sure to stay away
from these.

Dairy Food Bingers

Again, dairy food bingers often have extremely indi-
vidualized eating patterns. For instance, some binge
only on cheese, others binge exclusively on creamy

salad dressings, and still other dairy food bingers over-eat *anything* that contains milk.

For that reason, you will have to be brutally honest with yourself when deciding what to eat at fast-food, as well as at other, restaurants. The most common dairy product at these establishments is, of course, cheese. In addition, fast-food places use dairy-based condiments such as mayonnaise, butter, sour cream, milk-based salad dressings and hamburger sauces made with mayonnaise. If any of these foods trigger binges in you, then it's important to avoid them.

JAPANESE RESTAURANTS

My husband, who is Japanese-American, is infatuated with the cooking of his mother's native land. Since he's constantly pulling me into Japanese restaurants, I've learned to develop an avid appetite for Japanese food.

Since the Japanese use plenty of fresh vegetables in all their meals, Yo-Yo Syndrome sufferers can find many safe foods in a Japanese restaurant.

Bread Bingers

Be sure to avoid the noodles that come in a variety of Japanese food, such as sukyaki (a soup). Also pass up any foods that have a tempura batter, along with won-tons or egg rolls of any kind. Some bread bingers find themselves binging on rice; if rice is one of your binge foods, stay away from sushi, norimaki and any other rice dishes.

There are, fortunately, many foods in Japanese restaurants that bread bingers can enjoy. Among these are teriyaki beef or chicken, and stir-fries.

Sugar Bingers

There are few Japanese foods containing sugar, so you won't have much to worry about at these restaurants, with the exception of the obvious dessert foods. Some Japanese sauces, including teriyaki, plum and barbecue, contain sugar, and since even these small amounts can trigger binges, you'd do best to stay away from sauces of any kind (unless you can determine that they're sugar-free).

Salty Junk Food Bingers

Again, your task is to avoid the crispy fried foods such as tempura, noodles and a Japanese equivalent of trail mix containing dried peas and crackers. However, this represents such a small percentage of the typical Japanese restaurant fare that you'll find a large variety of foods to choose from.

Spicy Food Bingers

Since most Oriental food has a mild and even flavor, you're not likely to binge on anything in a Japanese restaurant. The exception could be food smothered with *wasabi,* or Japanese horseradish, so stay clear of this condiment. This pale green, pasty spice is usually offered on the side of sushi dishes and is fairly easy to avoid.

Dairy Food Bingers

Dairy foods are rarely offered in Japanese restaurants and I've seen only two Japanese dishes topped with white sauce—one was an Oriental version of chicken stroganoff and the other was a cold vegetable plate with a ranch-style dressing on it. Of course, most Japanese places offer ice cream, but basically dairy food bingers can relax when ordering in these restaurants because it's unlikely that they'll run into dairy products.

BARBECUE RESTAURANTS

No longer confined to summertime or limited to the backyard grill, barbecue-style food has found its way into some outstanding specialty restaurants. In Los Angeles, the better barbecue restaurants are always filled with patrons and the waiting time to be seated is upwards of an hour. I suspect this phenomenon isn't limited to the West Coast, either, because barbecued food seems to appeal to everyone.

Barbecued food, as with most food, fits right into the Yo-Yo Syndrome Diet, provided, of course, that you follow your eating plan. Watch out for fatty cuts of meat, especially on steaks and ribs, and remember the guideline about limiting red meat to once a week or less.

Bread Bingers

Most bread bingers will find barbecue restaurants contain plenty of food that they can eat without worry. The exceptions are biscuits, buns, onion rings, and breaded foods, and for most bread bingers, french fries and potato chips. Many barbecue restaurants also serve corn on the cob, a food that triggers binges in some bread bingers.

What *can* be enjoyed are any of the barbecued meats on the menu, such as chicken, ribs or steak. You can also have barbecued or baked beans and cole slaw along with your meal.

Sugar Bingers

Barbecue sauce, almost without exception, contains a lot of sugar. For this reason—unless you can be absolutely sure that the sauce is sugarless—you may want to avoid barbecue restaurants altogether. The alternatives to this include taking the skin off the barbecued chicken, ordering a meal without barbecue sauce, or eating items on the menu that normally aren't smothered with sauce (such as potatoes, rice or salad). Watch out for hidden sources of sugar in the barbecued beans, baked beans or cole slaw. But wouldn't it be easier to avoid this situation and eat at a different type of restaurant?

Salty Junk Food Bingers

Many salty junk food bingers go on eating binges when they eat crispy chicken skin, so either you'll want to avoid eating chicken or else remove the skin before eating it. Your best bet, instead, would be to order barbecued steak since it doesn't have the texture that can set off an eating binge.

Of course, you'll need to stay away from the fried, crispy side dishes often offered at barbecue restaurants, such as potato chips, french fries and onion rings. As an alternative, stay with barbecued or baked beans and cole slaw.

Spicy Food Bingers

Like the sugar binger, you may want to consider eating at another restaurant to avoid the prominence of your binge food in barbecue restaurants. Barbecue sauce is essentially equated with spiciness, so why set yourself up needlessly?

However, like the sugar binger, you can successfully eat around your binge food at a barbecue restaurant if you order chicken and remove the skin before eating. Or, you could order a steak grilled *without* sauce. Stay away from all barbecue sauce and barbecued beans. Baked beans, if they're not made with hot peppers, are a safe choice, as is cole slaw. In addition, you can enjoy biscuits and corn on the cob.

Dairy Food Bingers

There's very little dairy food at barbecue restaurants, with the exception of butter, biscuits (which are made with dairy products) and cole slaw (which is made with mayonnaise).

Other than these foods, you should be able to enjoy anything on the menu: barbecued meats, beans, rice, and unbuttered corn.

FRENCH RESTAURANTS

French restaurants have an oddly paradoxical appeal. On the one hand, these restaurants are very elegant and formal. Yet there's an atmosphere of relaxation as well, one in which the waiters and waitresses encourage you to take your time and savor the meal. Everything's at once formal, yet at ease. And for many dieters, French food equals calories.

While it's true that the heavy sauces and fatty meats used in the preparation of many French dishes add up to a lot of calories, it doesn't mean that the Yo-Yo Syndrome sufferer has to avoid French restaurants forever! Remember, in the Yo-Yo Syndrome Recovery Program, we're not counting calories. We're only avoiding binge foods and keeping portions moderate. While I definitely wouldn't recommend having French food more than once a week because of its high fat content, you can relax and enjoy eating this cuisine and not worry about gaining weight.

Since most French meals begin with a soup, I want to begin this discussion with a reassurance that every Yo-Yo Syndrome sufferer—regardless of his or her binge food—is able to eat the clear French stocks because they don't contain *any* bingeable ingredients. That's right—no sugar, flour, dairy products or intense spices! These clear soups (not the opaque or creamy ones) are often called *fond blanc* on the menu, as in *fond blanc de volaille* (chicken soup), *fond blanc de boeuf* (beef soup) and *fond blanc de veau* (veal soup).

Bread Bingers

As long as you pass up the bread and biscuits at the restaurant, you should find plenty of dishes to eat. Most main courses center on meat and vegetables smothered in sauces. Unlike other ethnic sauces, most French sauces aren't thickened with flour or cornstarch. However, because this is such an important point—since even the smallest amount of flour can send the bread binger into a compulsive overeating episode—be sure to ask your waiter or waitress about the preparation of any sauces before ordering. If the sauces are made with flour or cornstarch, then ask that your meal be prepared without sauce.

Any of the meat-with-vegetable dishes will fit into your Yo-Yo Syndrome Recovery Plan quite well.

Foods for you to avoid include soufflés, noodle dishes (*fraiches*), caviar that is served on toast or crackers, pâtés and meat loaves (which are prepared with flour), crêpes, and creamy soups thickened with flour.

Sugar Bingers

Like the bread binger, you'll find plenty of foods in a French restaurant that dovetail with your Yo-Yo Syndrome Recovery Plan—provided you stay clear of the dessert cart.

Exceptions to this are foods prepared with sweet sauces such as duck with orange sauce (*canard à l'orange*) and crêpes (which have sugar in their batter).

Try to stick with dishes that have creamy sauces, as opposed to fruit-based sauces to avoid any hidden sources of sugar. Ask the waiter or waitress, also, about the preparation of any vegetable side dishes—many French restaurants candy their carrots, peas or chestnuts. Your best choice will be a poultry or seafood dish.

Salty Junk Food Bingers

Since most French cooking involves roasted meats, the only foods you're likely to run into trouble with are fried, crunchy side dishes. These usually involve potatoes—after all, it was the French who gave us *pommes frites*—french fries. Variations on the french fry theme have all sorts of names, *pommes frites pont neuf* (short french fries), *pommes allumettes* (matchstick potatoes, or long french fries), *pommes gaufrettes* (similar to potato chips), *pommes soufflées* (puffed and fried potato slices) and *pommes pailles* (crispy potato noodles).

Other foods that, because of their crunchiness, may trigger a binge include crêpes, toast and potato gratin or sliced potatoes baked with cheese (*gratin de pommes de terre*).

With the exception of these and other crispy or fried foods, salty junk food bingers can feel free to order anything on the menu. Bon appétit!

Spicy Food Bingers

French food usually has a mild, but interesting intensity to it, so the spicy food binger probably won't run into anything in a French restaurant that would trigger an overeating episode. I have to say "probably" because each restaurant, of course, comes up with its own creations. But all in all, I'd say that French food is not intense or spicy enough to trigger a binge in you.

Therefore, you can relax and savor any of the delicious meals offered to you.

Dairy Food Bingers

Alas, poor dairy food binger! There's not much food available for you in a French restaurant. In fact, it'd be best for you to stay clear of all French restaurants because of the predominance of your binge food in these establishments. Almost *everything* is smothered in sauces made with plenty of heavy cream, eggs and real butter! And there are plenty of dishes that use cheese as an ingredient, as well.

Instead of listing the foods you should avoid, which is so unfortunately extensive, I'll list some suggestions for foods you can eat if you do go to a French restaurant. First, you can relax when the clear soup arrives at your table, because unless the soup is white or opaque, it doesn't contain any dairy products. Second, you can eat any salads (provided the dressing is a non-dairy variety, such as vinaigrette).

For a main course, your choices are limited to meats, rice and vegetables *without* creamy sauces. This means looking carefully at the menu or asking the waiter or waitress for a dish not prepared with cream, butter or eggs; for instance, meat prepared with *poivrade* (pepper) sauce (oil, wine, pepper and herbs). One such dish is roast leg of venison with poivrade sauce (*gigue de chevreuil à la sauce poivrade*), which is made without a trace of dairy products.

Another alternative is to ask to have the white sauce left off of your meal during its preparation; however, I can't guarantee what kind of reception you'll get for this request from the restaurant staff. Also, many French dishes are prepared with cream and butter *in* them as well as *on* them. In these cases, of course, leaving the sauce off the top of the meal won't eliminate the dairy products.

Finally, you can always peek at the back pages of the menu to see if the restaurant offers "American" (i.e., sauceless) dishes.

★   ★   ★

All in all, dining out should be fun and relaxing, and you needn't worry about your weight and Yo-Yo Syndrome Diet if you follow the guidelines in this chapter. In the next chapter, we'll look at how you can keep your diet intact in other situations where you might be vulnerable to overeating: on vacations, at parties, at work and with potentially pushy people.

11

Taking Your Yo-Yo Syndrome Diet out into the Real World

THERE'S NO doubt about it. Dieting is a lot of work, often requiring tremendous commitment in the face of temptation. There's the dessert cart the waitress pushes under your nose. The birthday cake at work. Aunt Mary's homemade chocolate chip cookies. And the tempting buffets of exotic foods offered on cruise ships. Sometimes it feels as if the whole world is ganging up on you, in one big effort to get you to abandon your diet! What's a dieter to do?

This chapter focuses on ways to keep your Yo-Yo Syndrome Diet on course, despite roadblocks and hurdles that invariably pop up on vacation, at work, during the holidays and at home. Just as you can improve your chances of surviving a fire unscathed by planning an escape route ahead of time, you can benefit from learning how to avoid these common dieting traps.

Tips on Traveling Without Overeating

The guidelines for restaurants given in Chapter 10 should be used while you're traveling or on vacation. In fact, it would be a good idea to pack this book in your suitcase for reference while you're away from home.

Most people complain of gaining weight while they're on vacation, and there are lots of reasons why this is so.

The first is that a lot of us have unrealistic expectations about how we'll feel before we go on vacation. Consider the couple, for instance, who saves for ten years and dreams of the day when they can go on a cruise to the Bahamas. The wife fantasizes about feeling elegant as she dines with the captain and dances in her evening gowns, while the husband dreams about lolling about on the deck and taking long snoozes in the afternoon sun.

Since the husband and wife have different mental pictures and expectations—all of which are sure to fall short of reality—they're likely to feel somewhat let down, frustrated and angry while they're on the cruise. After all those years of saving money and dreaming, they may feel cheated when the actual cruise doesn't match their fantasies.

And since cruise ships are notorious for offering round-the-clock buffets, how do you think Mr. and Mrs. Disappointed will spend their time? They're likely to stuff their disappointment with all-you-can-eat meals.

In the same vein, the busy executive who dreams all year of the two weeks in July when he can relax in Maui, may also be setting himself up for an eating binge. Once he gets to the Hawaiian island, he may feel as keyed-up as he does at the office, so he Stress Eats to try to relax. Or he finds that the crowds of tourists are extremely unrelaxing and tries to unwind and escape the stressors by overindulging in the restaurants that line the island shores.

Our unmet expectations about vacations can lead to disappointment, anger (especially with one's spouse), anxiety, frustration, and depression—all feelings that place us at high risk for Emotion Eating. Because of this, it's important to not look forward to your vacation *unrealistically*. Try not to look at your trip as a magical cure-all for all your stresses and problems. Basically, you will be the same person on your vacation with the same body and personality. Not that much will change, except for the scenery.

Yes, vacations are wonderful. But they're better when you keep your expectations for them down-to-earth and basic. Dream about being able to get away from phones and from work. Look forward to the pretty vistas you'll encounter. And yes, you'll probably be able to relax and have some fun, too. And by keeping your sights about the vacation a tad lower, you won't trigger the fattening feelings that lead Emotion Eaters to overeat.

The second major reason why vacations lead to overeating is the fatigue that accompanies travel and erratic schedules. If you travel by plane to another time zone, drive hundreds of miles, sleep in strange quarters, or party all night, your body's going to let you know that it's tired. And, as you may remember from Chapter 3, being tired—fat-igue—is the second most common feeling leading to Emotion Eating. We try to boost our energy by eating, when what we really need is sleep.

For this reason, it's a good idea to plan your vacation so that you're able to rest and relax as much as possible. Plan your arrival so that you can nap for an hour or two after checking in to the hotel. Don't expect to drive more hours than your body can withstand. Try to stay in hotels with comfortable accommodations. And don't abuse your body by staying up all night or overindulging in alcohol. Taking these measures will help you withstand the temptation to Emotion Eat or Stress Eat.

Another factor in vacation-time overeating is having more time and opportunity than normal to eat. Someone who's not used to relaxing, for instance, may feel uncomfortable with all the unstructured time of the vacation and try to fill the time with food-related activities: reading about the local restaurants, planning where to go for dinner that evening, calling to make reservations, dressing for dinner, driving to the restaurant and then, of course, eating the dinner. This alone can use up hours in a day.

And since you're not stuck at the office while on vacation, you'll have more time to spend eating. And the more time available, the greater the chance that the meal will be huge. Perhaps at work you have only 45 minutes to eat, and most of this time is spent getting to the restaurant. This means you'll only have time to grab a quick meal, such as a sandwich, before dashing back to the office. On vacation, however, every meal can last for hours . . . and hundreds more calories.

People who go on cruises get even more extra "opportunities" to overeat, because most cruises serve all-you-can-eat buffets several times a day. Those Yo-Yo Syndrome sufferers who worry about getting their money's worth, or who feel anxious about missing something, may fall into the trap of binging their way through the Caribbean.

In addition, many Snowball Effect Eaters overindulge on vacation because they confuse eating with entertainment. They think of gorging on food as part of the fun of traveling, and end up overeating in this misguided "recreation"; but they end up feeling fat instead of elated. Finally, vacations often end in disastrous weight additions because Binge Eaters eat their binge foods.

Your vacation probably comes just once a year, maybe even less often. It should be a happy, memorable time in your life. By staying on the Yo-Yo Syndrome

Diet during your travels, you'll feel better physically and emotionally.

Here are some tips, then, to keep in mind during your travels:

- Don't give up your exercise program while on vacation. While you may not have access to the same type of exercise equipment or setting you have at home, be sure to engage in some sort of physical activity every day. Try something new and fun such as dancing, swimming, tennis or racquetball. This will have several benefits, including:

  Keeping your muscles toned

  Burning calories

  Reducing fattening feelings and stress

  Providing healthy, non-caloric fun and entertainment

  Helping maintain your motivation for dieting

  Helping you feel good about your physical appearance

  Helping you keep your energy level higher

  Providing structured time, thereby reducing the chances that you'll eat out of boredom.

- Continue to plan your meals ahead of time. You can do this, even when you're on vacation, by reading the menu of the restaurant you plan to go to (usually found in hotel publications, travel guide magazines and on display in front of the restaurant) before you get inside the restaurant. Decide on a meal that fits your Yo-Yo Syndrome Diet before you sit down in the restaurant, so that impulsiveness doesn't cause you to go off your diet.

If you're eating at a buffet, use the guidelines given in Chapter 10: walk around the entire buffet first and note what looks good to you and what foods fit your Yo-Yo Syndrome Diet. Then choose up to six items that will fulfill your serving count for foods from the dairy, starch, meat, and fruit/vegetable groups for that meal. And remember the guideline of one serving only.

- Sightseers and vacationers traveling by car must be especially alert to stay on their diets. In an effort to conserve time and money, many car travelers cut corners at mealtime, and this can be disastrous for a diet! The following tips will help keep you on track:

First, if most of your meals are eaten at fast-food restaurants, try to stick to salads to avoid overdoing fatty fried foods and red meats. Second, avoid keeping snacks in the car, as the distractions of driving make many people overeat without realizing it. Instead, eat your snacks right after lunch and dinner so that they're more controlled. Finally, get out of the car for fresh air and exercise at least twice a day to keep your energy level up and reduce "fat-igue."

- Airplane travelers can reduce their chances of over-eating by taking two important steps: First, because food served on airlines is often greasy and difficult to digest during air travel, it's best to call the airline ahead of time and request a vegetarian meal or a fruit and cheese platter (something that almost all airlines are more than happy to provide). A special meal will contain fewer calories and make you feel more refreshed when you arrive at your destination.

  Second, plan your meals according to your destination's time zone. When traveling to a different time zone, it's easy to get mixed up about whether it's time for breakfast, lunch or dinner. On one trip I took before I was on my Yo-Yo Syndrome Diet —when I was still yo-yoing—I ate breakfast *before* driving to the airport for my 10 a.m. flight to Hawaii (which is 3 hours behind my state). When I was on the flight, the staff served breakfast, which I ate. Then, when I arrived at my hotel in Hawaii, it was 1 o'clock (island time), so I ate lunch. My body, though, tired from the flight and still accustomed to California time, felt as if it was dinnertime (4 p.m.). This meant I ate a larger than normal lunch. And that evening, I had a big dinner. Eating four large meals that first day of my vacation set me up to continue a food-centered holiday for my entire stay on Hawaii, and I gained 10 pounds in 11 days.

  To combat this now that I'm on the Yo-Yo Syndrome Diet, I plan my eating schedule ahead of time. If I'm taking a breakfast flight, I don't eat before going to the airport. I plan according to the time zone I'm traveling to, so I know *when and where* I'll be eating each meal. In this way, I reduce confusion about meal times and stick with my three meals a day.

- Plan your vacation itinerary around activities not involving food. Instead of making your restaurant trips the highlight of the day, center your day around a journey to a famous landmark. Or play a game with yourself or your companions about how much money you can save by eating light. Then, spend the extra money on a special non-food treat for yourself (such as a new outfit, theater tickets or a helicopter ride). You'll remember these treats a lot longer than you would another meal.

- Stress Eaters and Emotion Eaters must be sure to get enough relaxation and rest during their vacations. It's important to slow down from your normal hectic pace while you're on holiday. Guard against the habit of filling up each moment with activity, and allow for some lazing about and spontaneity during each day.

- Finally, it's extremely important that you continue weighing and looking at your naked body in a full-length mirror every day of your vacation. Otherwise, it's just too easy to lose sight of how much weight you may be gaining on vacation. I highly recommend packing a scale in your suitcase so that you always have one with you and to ensure that you have an *accurate* reading of your weight. If you don't have access to a full-length mirror in your hotel room or cabin, you may be forced to come up with creative means to examine yourself (such as crouching before a half-length mirror or standing on something to see your lower half in a standard bathroom mirror).

Food-filled Holiday and Birthday Survival Guide

Many Yo-Yo Syndrome sufferers have childhood memories of Christmases spent eating candies and Passovers and Thanksgivings filled with feasts. Holidays and food just seem to go hand-in-hand for most of us, making these times of the year very precarious when it comes to our eating and weight.

The emotional roller coaster that goes along with holidays can make this an especially difficult time of year for Emotion Eaters. There are feelings of loneliness from being away from your family on Christmas, grief because loved ones are no longer with you at Thanksgiving, sadness that you're no longer a child on Easter morning, and disappointment that your birthday wasn't remembered. Conversely, feelings of happiness and a desire to celebrate can also lead to food cravings for Emotion Eaters.

Holidays can be like vacations in that they are filled with unrealistic expectations. We may dream about the gifts we'll get on our birthday. And unconsciously, we may expect holidays to be similar to the ones we experienced as children. All these expectations set Emotion Eaters up for fattening feelings such as disappointment and emptiness.

For many of us, holidays mean "going home again," and there's a tendency to want to eat when you go to your parents' house. A friend of mine who's a Yo-Yo Syndrome sufferer, for instance, told me that the minute she sets foot in her parents' home (the same one she grew up in), she makes a beeline for the refrigerator. In looking at her reasons for doing this, she discovered that "going home" makes her feel like a little girl again. And as a little girl, she used to overeat a great deal. In other words, she has paired being home with eating Mom's cooking.

Ruth, a client of mine, tells me that her mother keeps candy in the same kitchen drawer today as she did when Ruth was a young girl. Every time Ruth goes home to visit her mother, she can barely keep from opening "the candy drawer" because it's such a powerful habit.

Still another client, Liz, tells me that when she goes home for the holidays, her mother frets over her by continually saying, "Liz, you're much too thin!" Then Liz's mother insists that she eat something, which Liz is more than happy to do since she loves her mother's baking.

The guidelines for eating during the holidays are the same as during any other day of the year. Your body, after all, never takes a day off from turning excess calories into body fat. Therefore, there's no special occasion to warrant overeating. Even if Grandma has prepared something especially for you.

I'm not being sarcastic when I say this. In my family, turkey dressing was a big deal, and Grandma Ada would lovingly prepare three different varieties every Thanksgiving. She'd make oyster stuffing, cornbread stuffing and sage stuffing—mmmm, I can taste them right now just writing this. Growing up, we'd all fight over the stuffings because we all loved the taste of them.

When I finally figured out that I binged every time I ate bread products, I feared what would happen on Thanksgiving when I turned down Grandma's three stuffings. And, at first, my family did resist the idea that I "couldn't eat bread anymore." I think they just humored me when they said "Okay." Besides, this way there was more stuffing for the rest of them.

I've since learned that it gets easier every year. And for the last several Thanksgivings, no one's even questioned why I don't eat stuffing with the rest of them. My family now accepts the fact that I don't eat sugar or bread. And that makes it infinitely easier for me to stay on my Yo-Yo Syndrome Diet during the holidays.

But not all families, of course, are as understanding as mine. In some households, you'd be insulting Grandma if you turned down some of her cooking, even if it was your binge food. What should you do in cases like this? Well, you could put a serving on your plate and then push it around with your fork so that it looks as if you've eaten some.

Or you could announce to your family that you've recently found you're allergic to this type of food (which is true—you break out in fat when you overeat). It would be difficult to dispute. After all, since you're an adult, your parents no longer keep tabs on your current medical condition. For all they know, you might break out in hives every time you eat sugar. You don't need to go into detail about the particular allergic reaction that occurs unless you believe doing so would be helpful.

Some of my clients have explained the Yo-Yo Syndrome Diet to their families and have found their explanations were met with great interest. One client, Debra, told me her family paid a great deal of attention to her as she explained the program last Christmas Eve—more attention than she had received in the past, and attention which she greatly enjoyed.

Each holiday is different, and in my clinic, we spend a great deal of time preparing clients to withstand every upcoming holiday. Some holidays, of course, are worse for some than they are for others. Here are some tips to help you stay thin through the holidays and birthdays:

- Yo-Yo Syndrome Sufferers often have a difficult time at Halloween, Easter, Passover, Hanukkah and Christmas when candy and desserts are pushed to such a strong degree. During these times, sugar bingers should take the following extra precautions:

  Don't *make* candy, baked goods or sweets to give as presents. This is a guaranteed way to make you overeat. Instead, give sugarless or non-food gifts.

When you're shopping, stay out of the candy aisles of the store so the sights and smells of the confections don't tempt you.

If Halloween candy is a temptation to you, then give trick-or-treaters non-food treats like nickels (which costs less than most candy!) or small, inexpensive plastic toys. Or pick a candy that you don't like and give that out.

Similarly, if making an Easter basket for your children spells t-e-m-p-t-a-t-i-o-n, or worse, a chocolate binge, then make Easter sugar-free for the kids from now on. For example, fill plastic eggs with money and hide them around your yard. Or fill the baskets with healthy treats (provided they're not a binge food for you) such as nuts, raisins, trail mix or hard-boiled eggs.

- Birthdays are another difficult time for Yo-Yo Syndrome sufferers, because someone will invariably bake a cake. How do you turn down a slice of cake that someone has bought or made especially for you? There are several solutions:

Let people know ahead of time that you can't eat any birthday cake. If you know they are going to buy or bake one for you, then politely tell them ahead of time "thank you but no thank you." I've found that this forewarning is appreciated, not resented. You could also suggest that the effort or money for the cake be used in other ways, such as for a light snack of diet gelatin or fruit salad. You could even create a new birthday tradition—and reduce pressures to overeat—by offering to be the person who'll pick up the tab for a low-calorie birthday lunch!

In a pinch, you can do as one of my clients did and take the cake graciously. But then go into another room, with no one watching, and dispose of the cake slice (via garbage disposal or trash can). Then you can easily turn down a second slice.

You could also use the old trick of mashing the cake around the plate with your fork, so that it appears you've eaten some. Another method is to throw a crumpled napkin over the cake slice, to both disguise it and create the appearance that you've finished eating.

- Probably your best defense against automatic eating triggered when you go home for the holidays is to prepare for it. For example, recall how your eating behavior changes when you go to your parents' (or other relatives') home. How can you plan to circumvent the pressure to eat there? If you're a Binge Eater, what steps can you take so that you won't eat your binge food while you're home?

  To avoid feeling like a little girl or boy (and thereby setting yourself up to overeat if you did so as a child), take some office or school work with you when you go to your parents. This "grown-up" material will provide a reminder of who you are as an adult; it will anchor you in the reality that you *are* an adult.

- Emotion Eaters need to guard against stuffing feelings during the holidays and on birthdays. These emotionally volatile occasions, as mentioned before, are ripe for triggering overeating episodes. Feel yourself burning with anger at the way Uncle Ed talks to you? Jealous because your sister's husband gave her diamonds for Christmas and you got a blender from your husband? Upset because Dad's drinking too much brandy when his doctor told him to knock off the liquor? If you don't feel you can talk about it without causing a major family rift at a very inopportune time, then be sure to get the anger out in other ways. Follow the guidelines outlined in Chapter 3 to stay on top of your fattening feelings: First, always admit your feelings to yourself instead of fighting or ignoring them. Second, help the troubling emotions subside by talking about them with a person who's nonjudgmental and a good listener, write your feelings out in private, or go for a walk and talk to yourself about your feelings. Third, don't overeat because of your fattening feelings—it'll only make you feel worse!

- If Thanksgiving dinner means you'll be nibbling before and after the meal *plus* eating three servings of a huge turkey banquet, then consider the following:

  Why not eat at a restaurant next year? That way, you won't be fat-igued from cooking all day. In addition, there will be no temptation to nibble while cooking, and no leftovers to worry about.

  If you do eat Thanksgiving at home, be sure to chew sugarless gum while you're cooking. Sampling food and chewing gum are two activities, fortunately, that don't go together simultaneously. In addition, keep a glass of water or iced tea handy and drink it instead of picking at the turkey dressing or whatever else you're preparing.

Plan ahead of time, as you normally do, what you'll be eating for Thanksgiving. Compose a personal menu that follows the Yo-Yo Syndrome Diet and vow to stick to it no matter what.

Be sure to eat breakfast and lunch on Thanksgiving Day. Starving before dinner serves no purpose other than to make you hungrier and more likely to overeat that night.

If you're the host or hostess, serve yourself last during dinner, so that by the time you sit down to eat, others will have had time to make a substantial dent in their meals. That way, the smaller portions on your plate won't stand out as radically different from the amount of food others have.

If someone asks you why you're not returning for seconds, hold your stomach and in your best Meryl Streep manner, say, "I'm absolutely stuffed! If I eat another bite, I swear I'll pop!" Few people will argue with you if you say this.

When others are filling up on pumpkin pie, keep your hands full by clearing the table, drinking some coffee or eating a Yo-Yo Syndrome Diet snack. If you can find it, buy yourself ahead of time a small carton of pumpkin-pie-flavored frozen yogurt—it's delicious and you won't feel so deprived!

Remember the true meaning of Thanksgiving involves gratitude, not food.

After dinner, send as many leftovers as you can home with guests to avoid overeating after dinner or the next day.

If this isn't possible, then divide the leftovers into small portions and put them in the freezer immediately. You won't be as likely to overindulge if the food isn't readily accessible.

- Many people postpone or put their diets on hold during the holidays. This is especially true of the time period from Thanksgiving through New Year's, when people tend to let the eating floodgates loose; on New Year's Eve, they resolve to bring the overeating season to a halt. This is a practice that many seasonal Snowball Effect Eaters are particularly likely to engage in. If you have this habit, remember that the Yo-Yo Syndrome Diet doesn't have a beginning or an ending. It is a way of life. Also keep in mind that your body doesn't take a holiday from converting calories into fat. It doesn't know whether today's your birthday or Christmas—it still gains or loses weight in the same way.

Wedding Receptions

How many of you have gone to a wedding reception or a party and then spent the majority of the evening parked next to the snack table? I know I have.

In my therapy practice, I've listened to more stories about overeating occurring at wedding receptions and parties than at any other place. And of these two, wedding receptions are definitely the number one place where Yo-Yo Syndrome sufferers go off their diets.

Many Yo-Yo Syndrome sufferers run into their fattening feelings at weddings. These may occur because you feel left out, feel that no one's paying attention to you, feel jealous that the bride's getting all the attention and gifts, feel aware of the contrast between your marriage and that of the bride-to-be's, or feel angry about being around drunk people and in close proximity to acquaintances or relatives whom you may not care for.

Sally, for example, was on the Yo-Yo Syndrome Diet for four months when she was invited to her cousin's wedding. The wedding was at a huge resort and the bride's parents spent a fortune on catering, flowers and wedding dresses. Sally was jealous of the money and attention her cousin, the bride, was getting but at the same time felt guilty for being petty. Sally also didn't know quite how to act at so regal an affair and felt very uncomfortable and self-conscious. She didn't know whether to fold her arms or keep her hands in her pockets as she stood at the wedding reception.

"Everyone else seems so sure of themselves," Sally thought. "They all fit in here, but I don't!" Feeling left out and sorry for herself, Sally headed toward the buffet table even though she knew the food would tempt her. She looked at the chocolate torte with the delicate roses frosted on each slice and thought, "One of those would make me feel better. I've lost fifteen pounds for this wedding and no one even noticed it. Just one piece of cake won't hurt me. No one will know . . . no one will even care!"

Before she could talk herself out of it, Sally had the torte in her mouth and was lovingly, almost sensuously, appreciating its creaminess. Too quickly, it was gone, and Sally unhappily grabbed another slice.

Sally felt nauseated with sugar and chocolate by the time she pulled herself away from the remaining slices of cake. Counting what was left—had she really eaten *that many?*—Sally felt disgusted with herself.

A wedding is an emotionally charged situation. It's very draining, whether you're in the audience or the wedding party, and the abundance of food afterward often spells trouble for the Yo-Yo Syndrome sufferer who feels in an emotional upheaval about the whole event. What can Yo-Yo Syndrome sufferers do to avoid going off their diets at a wedding?

First, stay as far away from snack tables as you can. This is particularly true if the event is being held at your own home or at a stranger's home, because at both places you're likely to feel anxious and pressured.

My client Jo, for instance, overate when she held a wedding reception at her house because she was so worried that the guests wouldn't approve of the job she had done in decorating and catering. Another client, Jeannie, went to a wedding where she didn't know anyone. Because she felt so self-conscious and awkward ("I was sure everyone knew I didn't know anyone there," she told me), Jeannie stood by the snack table all evening to appear busy. She ended up having her binge food that night and went on an all-out eating binge.

Second, go out of your way to mingle with others at the wedding. If you're uncomfortable because you don't know many people at the wedding, look for someone else who seems uncomfortable or lonely and ask them an open-ended question (one that can't be answered with a "yes" or a "no") such as, "How long have you known Tom and Mary?" "Whereabouts do you live?" or "What time is the band supposed to start playing?" If you don't get a positive reception to your question, find someone else to talk to.

Third, if you have some fattening feelings before, during or after the wedding, keep in mind you can choose to not go to the reception, or you can make a very brief appearance at it.

Parties and Get-Togethers

Parties, though they're meant to be fun occasions, can at times be extremely stressful, particularly if you're feeling fat and uncomfortable with the way you look. Feeling awkward with the people around you. Feeling invisible, as if you don't matter to anyone—or the opposite, feeling as if everyone's staring at you and judging you. All these feelings can send you to the chip and dip bowl, where you're apt to munch away your anguish instead of deal with it.

There also can be pressure to eat at parties. A friend of mine, for instance, throws the most elaborate parties. The trouble is, they all revolve around food and eating. As you walk into his house, the first sight you see is a giant oak table in an elevated dining room. The table is practically buckling under the weight of dozens of sterling silver platters, bowls and pitchers—all containing the most aesthetically appealing food you've ever seen. Guests spend most of the evening wandering around the table looking at the food, eating the food and talking about the food. At parties such as this, it's difficult to diet and remain inconspicuous.

However, instead of avoiding the company of my friend and the other guests, I've learned to follow the guidelines below to both have a good time *and* stay on my diet:

- The first, and most important, rule for staying on diets at parties is to eat your meal before going to the party. Make it a leisurely meal, complete with plenty of liquids to fill you up. Decide beforehand that you won't be eating anything at the party.

- Wear a snug belt around your waist to serve as a reminder to stay away from food.

- Weigh yourself before you leave to go to the party. This will keep your motivation for dieting high during the evening.

- Arrive fashionably late to the party. This way, the others will have already eaten so they won't be as apt to notice that you're not eating.

- Carry a glass of water, diet soda or white wine in your hand. This will reduce the risk of feeling awkwardly empty-handed, as well as prevent others from pushing plates of food into your hands.

- If the party is a potluck, picnic or barbecue, bring a low-calorie dish such as a colorful vegetable tray, fresh fruit salad or a bowl of sugar-free gelatin with fruit floating in it. That way, if you become desperate to eat, you'll have something to munch on that won't sabotage your dieting efforts.

- If you feel the urge to eat, quickly offer to help the host or hostess with party details. Pour drinks for other guests, fold napkins, take arriving guests' coats or drive to the store for some forgotten party necessity. Just do something other than eat!

- If you have any fattening feelings such as anger, embarrassment or jealousy, go into the nearest restroom or go outside alone. Close your eyes for a few moments and take three deep breaths. Tell yourself something comforting, such as "I'm a good person" or "I like myself." Give yourself a mental hug and when you feel composed, return to the party.

- If you're not having a good time, or if you feel out of control with your dieting willpower, then excuse yourself and leave the party. People leave parties early all the time; give yourself permission to do so if you need to.

Keeping Up the Diet at Work

Whether it's a cafeteria, the pastry cart, the co-worker's candy dish or the vending machine down the hall, temptations to overeat abound at the workplace. What's a Yo-Yo Syndrome sufferer, bent on losing weight, supposed to do? Let me tell you about some of the ingenious solutions my working clients have come up with.

Katherine keeps a pretty bowl of sugar-free hard candies and gum on her desk. She says that by keeping her mouth busy with sugarless treats, she keeps her mind off of the fattening foods her co-workers indulge in.

Patty was upset because there was always a big open box of doughnuts in the office lounge. Every time she'd take a break, the doughnuts would be right there staring her in the face. Now she throws a big towel over the box when she's on break—kind of an "out of sight, out of mind" way of dealing with it.

Sonya, who was faced with the same dilemma, solved it by talking with her co-workers and requesting that they keep the doughnut box up on a shelf where it was still accessible to others, but out of Sonya's sight.

In a similar situation, Hope worked in the back office of a grocery store and had a desk that faced a giant display of cookies. Every day, Hope stared at the cookies and sometimes did more than stare—she ate them! To conquer this problem, Hope finally had to change to a desk across the room.

Dale was perhaps in an even worse situation than Hope. She worked in a candy store! At first, Dale thought she might have to switch professions in order to keep her weight under control. But, instead, she decided to mentally "gross herself out" to stop the candy from tempting her. She imagines bugs walking across all the candy, bugs that leave a trail of insect debris. Dale's elaborate mental trick is very effective in making her appetite for candy go away.

Bridget's problem was that every time she'd get frustrated at work, she'd stomp away from her desk and head for the candy vending machine. Now that she's been on the Yo-Yo Syndrome Diet for three months, Bridget stomps off to the soda machine and buys a diet cola.

Margie, another client who was hooked on vending machine candy and chips, found there was only one way to keep herself away from this junk food: she stopped bringing any money to work.

Dianna solved the same problem in a different way. She explained to her close friends at work that she was trying to lose weight, and asked if they would please help her when she was about to break her diet. Luckily, Dianna's co-workers are good friends (you wouldn't want to make such a request to just anybody!), because they've given her support at times when she was just about to go off her diet. "Twice I've been walking down the hall toward the vending machines," Dianna told me, "and my friends have run up to me and said, 'Oh no you don't, Dianna! You're not going to break your diet now, not after you've lost this much weight!' " While we have to take responsibility ourselves for our dieting and eating, having support from others at work is definitely helpful.

Another client, Leigh, convinced her employer to start an exercise program for employees. The employer got Leigh and her co-workers a special group rate at a local gym, and this spurred many people in the company to become weight- and health-conscious. Now instead of sitting around eating pastries all day, the co-workers exchange diet tips and go to the gym together after work.

Mary has learned to schedule her workday so that

she's busy when her co-workers are snacking. While she still eats lunch with others, Mary plans her breaks so that the pastry cart is not around when she leaves her desk.

Sarah has found that she eats less and feels more satisfied if, after eating her Yo-Yo Syndrome Diet lunch, she takes a brisk walk around the high school where she teaches. Lately, she's been walking with another weight-conscious teacher, and it appears that Sarah's found herself a new friend in the process.

Tiffany was so fed up with having desserts pushed at her and left on her desk by co-workers that she decided to bring in a pepper shaker and keep it on her desk. Now whenever a pushy co-worker won't take "no" for an answer and insists on giving Tiffany some food, she pours pepper on it. This renders it inedible, removes the temptation, and shows her co-worker that she's serious when she says "No, thank you!"

Another client, Angela, had to admit to herself that she was encouraging her co-workers to push fattening goodies on her. Angela unwittingly was giving her co-workers a lot of attention every time she'd protest their offers of candy or cookies.

Elaine always seemed to be in a quandary every day on her lunch hour—should she eat lunch or run errands? There never seemed to be enough time to do both, and that meant Elaine would often skip lunch and overeat later, at dinnertime. Finally, Elaine had to examine her priorities. She clearly saw that skipping lunch was not a viable option for her if she wanted to maintain her weight loss. So Elaine has learned to run errands after work and on weekends.

Tom found that he'd unintentionally overeat when he worked through his lunch hour. To stop this tendency, Tom made a strict pact with himself to not eat at his desk.

Ruth, a Stress Eater, would overeat when she'd take potential clients out to lunch. Finally, Ruth had to figure out a way to stop this tendency without hurting her business. She's found that using relaxation techniques (outlined in Chapter 5) before a business lunch helps calm her nerves. She also limits her business lunches to one particular restaurant where foods on the Yo-Yo Syndrome Diet are served.

The cafeteria at the hospital where Jan worked rarely serves food that fits into her Yo-Yo Syndrome Diet. Most of the food on their menu consists of fatty meats covered with buttery sauces. To stay on the Diet, Jan had to start bringing her own lunches to work—something that requires extra planning, but is worthwhile in terms of Jan's success on the Diet. Sometimes she brings a "light," 300-calorie, frozen dinner and microwaves it at work. Other times, she'll prepare a Yo-Yo Syndrome chef's salad and keep it in the hospital kitchen's cafeteria until lunchtime.

Lisa couldn't stomach eating breakfast before going to work (she left at 6 a.m. to commute to work). She used to skip breakfast, but after beginning the Yo-Yo Syndrome Diet, she has begun making both her breakfast and lunch at night and bringing them to work with her the next day.

Audrey worked the 11 p.m. to 7 a.m. shift at a factory, and she found that the graveyard shift was not at all helpful in breaking out of her Yo-Yo Syndrome. It seemed Audrey was always mixed up about what time of day it was, and never knew whether it was time for breakfast, lunch or dinner (kind of like me when I travel to a different time zone on an airplane!). "I wake up at 9 p.m. to get ready for work and eat my first meal of the day," Audrey explained. "Now is that my breakfast because it's my first meal, or is it my dinner because I'm eating at 9 at night?" Unfortunately, this confusion often meant Audrey ate too much food, too many times a day. She'd also go right to sleep after eating in the late morning hours. Finally, Audrey had to admit that her graveyard shift was spelling the death of her dieting efforts. Her solution was to get transferred to the first shift (7 a.m. to 3 p.m.), and in this way, she was able to stick to her Yo-Yo Syndrome Diet and have three meals a day.

Carol learned not to tell her co-workers that she was dieting. "When I'd say I was on a diet, it was like I was a Buckingham Palace Guard the way they spent all their time taunting me and trying to tempt me with food so I'd go off my diet!" Once she kept this news to herself, her co-workers left her alone.

On Spouses, Lovers, Relatives and Friends

Carol's situation at work with taunting, teasing and tempting co-workers is probably similar to reactions you may have received while dieting. What do you do when you're dieting and one of the following happens to you?

Your spouse begins to bring home boxes of your favorite desserts.

Your mother insists you try the cake she baked just for you.

Your best friend says you look gaunt and "way too thin" (even though you really want to lose another 15 pounds).

Your sister asks for details about your diet plan, then proceeds to list reason after reason why "it'll never work for you."

Your boyfriend tells you he likes the way you look now, and insists he doesn't find thin women attractive.

Quite likely, you've met with these and similar situations that have either made you uncomfortable or proven to be a catalyst for overeating. It's also likely you'll have encounters like these in the future, so it's best to prepare for them in advance. This doesn't mean being defensive or carrying a chip on your shoulder; just having a few tools ready in case you need them.

As I mentioned in Chapter 6, it's important for you to understand exactly why you want to lose weight. If you're trying to slim down to garner compliments from your spouse or lover, then you've given him too much power over the course of your diet. You'll become discouraged when he doesn't notice the ten pounds you lost, and you'll feel you've been given "permission" to overeat if he gives you chocolate candies.

To maintain an attractive figure, the only motivating force that works is *losing weight to please yourself*. Unless you have the distorted body image that accompanies the eating disorder anorexia nervosa, you must adhere to your own standards of what weight feels best on you. If someone says you look like a skeleton and you still are above what the standard weight charts recommend for your height, then disregard the comment. Phrases like, "If you lose any more weight, you'll blow away" are meant to be flattering compliments, not a standard to determine whether you should go off your diet or not.

If people are pushy in their "you're too thin" admonishments, you can handle the situation in one of several ways: you can pretend you didn't hear them and change the subject or remain silent; you can thank them for the compliment and then change the subject; you can say, "Thanks for your concern, but I think I know best what weight I feel comfortable with. If I need some feedback in the future, I'll be sure to ask you for it"; or you can say (after repeated attempts to get the person to knock it off), "I feel distressed that you don't seem to hear me when I tell you to back off about my eating. I'm really growing to resent the intrusions, and I'm afraid if you don't stop that it'll hurt our relationship."

But what about the people who push food under your nose, sending delicate vapors directly into your brain's appetite center? What about the man who three months ago teased you about the size of your behind but is now offering you bites of his candy bar? And how about your poor Mama, who seemingly slaved to create the fattening dessert she's now pushing on you? Could you ever live with yourself again if you turned *her* down?

What should you do in these admittedly slippery situations? If you know you're likely to encounter a diet saboteur, then your best bet is to psyche yourself up the same way you would for any challenging situation, such as asking your boss for a raise.

As you're getting dressed to go to Mom's for dinner, mentally rehearse how you will keep your diet intact for the evening. Remember, you are an adult and how you eat *is your business, and nobody else's!* When you say "no" to someone's offering, you are not rejecting that person; you are rejecting the food in his or her hands.

Try to put yourself in the other person's shoes to understand what is motivating him or her to push food on you. Everyone's not out to get you, even though it can feel that way at times. For example, one client I had complained that her husband brought home her favorite doughnuts every night. At first, she was furious that he could be so insensitive.

Upon looking more closely at her situation, however, we found that she was actually rewarding her husband for bringing home doughnuts. She'd act very happy, agreeable and loving the whole time she was eating the doughnuts, and this attitude encouraged her husband to bring home the pastries every night.

Be assertive and spell out exactly how you feel about their food pushing. Assertiveness, unlike aggressiveness, means that you have regard for the other person's feelings while you talk about your own feelings. For instance, an aggressive person would say, "I'm so mad at you for bringing home those damn cookies when I've asked you not to! How could you be so stupid?"

An assertive person, in contrast, would phrase the same feelings in a way that would permit communication because defensiveness would be kept to a minimum. A better way of expressing anger might sound something like this: "I need to tell you that I feel exasperated right now. I am trying really hard to lose weight, and it's a very difficult thing to do. What I need right now more than anything is your support, and that means not bringing the cartons of ice cream home with you at night. Please stop, okay? I really mean this—it's important to me."

Unless the other person truly has some hidden reasons for wanting to sabotage your diet, saying something assertive like this should bring an end to the problem. If not, try to have a discussion about what's *really* going on, because it would probably mean jealousy's at the root of it all.

When Others Become Jealous

Roberta came into my office and started crying. "I feel so guilty!" she sobbed. "My husband is sure that I'm going to have an affair now that I've lost the weight, and I hate to see him so upset and worried." Roberta had no intent of cheating on her husband, but she did want to protect him from his emotional pain. She was seriously considering putting her weight back on just to regain peace in her house. Fortunately, she talked herself out of it, realizing that *she'd* be miserable if she were overweight again.

Roberta's spouse, like many husbands, did initially feel threatened when his wife transformed into a svelte beauty. He felt insecure, as if he were unworthy of being married to such an attractive woman. Surely she would now leave him for a man befitting her.

Only time heals the spouse's insecurities. When your husband, boyfriend, wife or girlfriend sees that you are not going to leave, he or she will relax. If he or she doesn't, you will next have to look at your own behavior to be certain you are not provoking the jealousy (by flaunting flirtations in front of him or her, for instance). If you aren't doing anything to warrant the jealousy, then you'll need to conclude that your lover has a personal problem with insecurity and if this is the case, you may not be able to change him or her into a secure person. Deep insecurity—the kind that doesn't respond to reassurances from others—often has its roots in earlier experiences with rejection (from parents or a first love, for example) and so has nothing to do with you.

Your best bet in dealing with a spouse or lover who displays jealousy is an honest exchange of feelings about one another. You can begin such a talk with sharing your own deep feelings. Choose a quiet moment when you're alone together and uninterrupted for a while and begin with something like, "I feel there have been some changes in the way we relate to one another lately, and it all seems to have happened since I lost weight. It really upsets me, too, and I wonder if we could talk about it." Avoid hurling accusations. Don't say anything like "You seem so jealous lately," as this is apt to be met with defensiveness and denial.

The response to your opening statement will likely sound something like, "Yeah, I know there've been some changes! You sure have changed since you lost the weight!"

Even though your jaw may fall open at this moment, resist the impulse to defensively say, "Me? You think *I'm* the one who's changed?!" Instead, ask your lover for more information to get to the heart of his or her jealousy: "In what ways do you see that I've changed?" You may be surprised by his or her answer, but you'll probably hear the truth.

At this point, share all of your feelings with your lover. Tell him or her what being thin and changing your life means to you. Talk about how exciting your life is now, and how you'd like to see your lover work on some life-enriching goals, too. And most of all, reassure your lover that all of these changes do not spell rejection. You are not leaving him or her, you're just shedding your fat lifestyle.

Again, it may take time for your lover to adjust to the new you. Stick with it, though, and don't go back to your old body no matter how jealous the other person becomes. No one is worth your being overweight again.

Not only lovers become jealous. Your same-sex friends may become jealous when your body starts to slim down. As a result, you may experience fears of

rejection, abandonment, anger at their conditional love
and hurt at being excluded.

At first Charlotte thought she was imagining being
excluded from the parties and get-togethers that her
small circle of friends customarily engaged in. "For
years, Harry and I would meet with three other couples
for drinks, dinner or card games," Charlotte told me.
"We were all really close and enjoyed each other's company tremendously!" That is, until Charlotte lost 30
pounds.

"I had always been struggling with my weight," she
explained, "but I'd been heavy since these people had
known me. When I decided to diet, they were all so
supportive! They complimented me on the way I
looked each time they saw me, and after I got the whole
thirty pounds off, they made me feel like a princess. I
mean, a couple of the husbands in the group kept staring at me all evening." Charlotte's eyes turned downward. "It's painful to think about—and I think it really
sounds vain of me—but I'm sure that two of the gals in
our group are jealous of me now, and that's why they
haven't invited Harry and me to the get-togethers for
the past month."

Another client, Sandra, was also stinging from the
pain of rejection connected to her weight loss. Her circle
of friends had consisted of five other women she'd
known from church, who went out to lunch twice a
week together. They'd eat enormous meals, complete
with dessert, and spend hours talking about their kids,
their husbands and life in general.

When Sandra first began to diet, the others teased her

with "ah, you'll never do it!" gibes. Then, as Sandra continued to eat small lunches and pass up dessert, the comments turned into cold shoulders. "I could feel that they were mad at me," Sandra remembered. "It was like I was violating some code of ethics by dieting." The group's attitude became so uncomfortable for Sandra that she began missing the lunch dates and avoiding the group members at church. The ensuing feelings of loneliness and betrayal almost sent Sandra back to overeating more than a few times.

When a friend signals jealousy over your weight loss, it's important to remember a few things. First, the bad feelings your friend is experiencing aren't coming from you, they're coming from within that person. I remember one summer when I was carrying 35 extra pounds on my body. It was a hot summer, and I spent a lot of time at my sister-in-law's swimming pool where we had a great time splashing about (she and I were both overweight). Some days, though, her cousin—a tall, thin clotheshorse—would join us at the pool. Between her body and her wardrobe, I remember *despising* that cousin. She was a nice person, and never did one mean thing to me, but when I saw her I felt bad about myself. And instead of acknowledging those feelings, I transferred them onto her.

Second, if your jealous friends have always been close to you, then have a heart-to-heart talk with them just as you would with a spouse or lover (as described above). And remember, a *true* friend will love you whether you're fat or thin. If someone rejects you because of what you look like, he or she wasn't a very good friend to begin with.

Finally, if the jealous friend was just a superficial acquaintance, then it may be time to let go of the relationship. You don't need to waste precious moments of your life trying to please someone who doesn't have your best interests at heart. And if this person threatens your diet by triggering fattening feelings in you, you especially need to avoid him or her.

It's a cliché, but it's so true and especially appropriate in this discussion on dealing with others: You can't please everyone, but you can please yourself. Losing weight and dieting is not a thoughtless act that can hurt someone you care about. It's not selfish in the usual sense of the word. Therefore, it's illogical for others to treat you badly as you lose weight. While you should try to understand their point of view, you shouldn't let anyone step on you. Take good care of yourself through your Yo-Yo Syndrome Diet and be your own best friend.

Ending on a Friendly Note

Not everyone will have ulterior motives or be jealous as you lose weight. Some social obstacles are created by practical sources. Think for a moment about when and where you normally see your friends. Chances are you'll answer, "When we eat dinner together." Many people who diet give up these social gatherings, and along with them, the chance to be with their friends.

However, there are lots of ways to maintain your social network and not be inviting disaster for your Yo-Yo Syndrome Diet. Among them:

- Have a Yo-Yo Syndrome Diet party! Why not throw a party for you and your friends and serve meals from the Yo-Yo Syndrome Diet menu? Even your friends who aren't dieting will appreciate the opportunity to get together and will enjoy your lighter, more natural foods.

  Parties can also revolve around some activity other than eating. How about a horseshoe throw or a swimming party? Why not organize a painting party, where everyone comes dressed in their grub- bies and pitches in to get a whole house painted in an afternoon? Offer organized games such as cha- rades for your guests, or hire a band and clear the floor for some calorie-burning dancing. How about a sing-along around the piano? (Sounds corny, I know, but it really is fun!) At a party with a non- food theme, you and your guests will have fun and welcome the change from stuffy sit-down dinner parties.

- Exercise with your friends. Don't see much of your friends now that you don't go out to lunch with them anymore? Why not invite one or two of them to go to the gym with you? Or buy your best friend a one-month, half-year or full-year membership at the gym you attend for her birthday.

Another great idea is to form a walking group. Decide on a time and meeting place and then go for long walks with your friends. This will give you lots of time to catch up on the latest news, expose you to fresh air and pretty scenery, and help burn those calories.

- Go shopping for new clothes with your friends. Whether you buy, window-shop or just try on different styles, clothes shopping is a good way to stay inspired to lose weight or maintain your goal weight. Shopping with friends can turn an average shopping day into a fun adventure. And be sure to visit the swimsuit department—it'll really motivate you to get or stay slim!

- Sign up for a fun class with a friend. Have you ever had a secret yearning to learn how to make stained glass windows, go windsurfing, or improve your photography skills? Chances are that one or two of your friends have, too. Why not check the schedule of the local adult school, the parks and recreation department or the community college nearest you? After getting the necessary information, urge your interested friends to enroll with you. Not only will you get to spend time together in an activity that doesn't involve food, you'll also have fun and learn new skills.

Dieting doesn't have to mean isolating yourself from people whose company you enjoy. You still can eat lunch or dinner together, after all, as long as you stick with your Yo-Yo Syndrome Diet menu (it's even easier and more fun if your friends are also on the Yo-Yo Syndrome Diet). I think you'll find that the longer you stay on the Diet, the more you'll want to spend your free time playing, learning, and generally being active. You won't want to spend all your time eating anymore!

12

Keeping the Weight off for Good: Maintenance Measures

MANY OF US, raised on a steady diet of fairy tales and happily-ever-after bedtime stories, are unconsciously looking for easy, magical solutions to our problems. We want results, and we want them now!

While the thought of magical interventions makes for nice endings in Mother Goose stories, in real life, of course, we have to work at making our lives happier. No Prince Charming or fairy godmother is going to make our fat cells shrink. No magical unicorn is going to reduce our waistlines. And no new diet book, gym or diet club, in and of itself, is going to make us lose weight either. That's the bad news.

The good news, though, is this: If you've decided you've wasted enough years gaining and losing weight on your Yo-Yo Syndrome, you can use the steps of the Diet and change all that forever. You can lose weight and never gain it back again.

One Day at a Time, One Pound at a Time

Each step of the Yo-Yo Syndrome Recovery Program is equally important, and all need to be followed in order for permanent weight loss to be achieved. As this book has discussed, the road to weight loss is fraught with emotional and environmental roadblocks, and you need commitment and motivation to stay on track.

One of the best ways to keep your commitment and motivation up is by making a contract with yourself and putting your goals in writing. In my therapy practice, I have clients complete and sign a contract just like the one printed here. It's a powerful tool, and I highly recommend that you use it for yourself. Every one of my clients tells me that, after they signed the contract, they didn't even consider breaking it; after all, they had promised me that they'd do everything listed in it.

An important component of the contract is that it is

signed by a witness. All Yo-Yo Syndrome sufferers have made promises to themselves such as "I'll stick to my diet today" only to break the promises within days or minutes of making them. I've found that Yo-Yo Syndrome sufferers almost always break promises made to themselves, but almost compulsively *keep* promises made to others. Most Yo-Yo Syndrome sufferers, for example, are extremely punctual, and if they promise to be somewhere at 3 p.m., they will break their necks to be there on time.

This characteristic is why your weight contract should be signed by a witness. Think of it as a way to promise someone else that you're going to follow the measures outlined on the contract. You'll still be losing weight to please yourself, but during those moments when your taste buds hanker for something fattening, it'll be easier to stick to your diet if you remember, "Oh yes, I promised so-and-so I wouldn't overeat."

Choose your witness carefully, though. It must be someone you can confide in and someone with whom you share a relationship based on mutual respect. Someone who is caring and nonjudgmental. Someone who won't tease or taunt you about your weight or diet. It could be your spouse, friend, co-worker, therapist, parent, professor, physician, exercise instructor or child—anyone. The important thing is not to put off completing your contract.

To complete your contract, photocopy it from this book and then use ink to complete and sign it. Have someone who is loving and nonjudgmental (and preferably, someone who is also recovering from the Yo-

Yo Syndrome) witness the contract by signing it below your name. In this way, you're less likely to break the terms of the contract. After you're finished, hang the contract in a prominent location—the best place is the refrigerator or pantry door—as a reminder that you've promised to stick with the steps of the Diet.

There's no better time than now to have a body you're proud of. How many more summers do you want to slip by before you get into shape? How many more Christmas parties do you want to feel fat at? How about high school reunions? Wouldn't you like to feel trim and svelte at your next one?

And even more importantly, wouldn't you like to feel good about yourself and your life? Wouldn't you like to wake up in the morning and feel excited as you look forward to the day's events?

There's no better time to begin working toward your goals than today. After all, tomorrow will be pretty much like today. There's no reason not to start taking steps toward transforming your life and your body in ways that'll make you happy . . . *now*.

If, during the months or years following your signing of the Yo-Yo Syndrome Diet Contract, you do happen to slip, don't give up on yourself. Instead, photocopy another contract, promptly sign it and start over again.

If you do slip, don't kick yourself or say, "I'm a failure." Such negative talk only leads into the downward emotional spirals that keep you overeating. My mother, who is a recovering Yo-Yo Syndrome sufferer, has a great way of demonstrating this:

Let's say you're driving from your house to the air-

The Yo-Yo Syndrome
Diet Contract

I, _____, hereby
contract with myself to lose weight. My present weight
is _____ and my ideal weight is _____.
At the rate of losing between 8 to 16 pounds per month,
it will take me between _____ and _____ months
to lose my excess weight.

Today, I promise to do the following in order to lose
weight: Follow the steps of the Yo-Yo Syndrome Diet
(check all that apply):

Eat according to the Yo-Yo Syndrome Diet guidelines.

Binge Eaters: Abstain from my binge foods, which are:

_____

_____

_____

Emotion Eaters: Wait 15 minutes after feeling hungry,
and deal with my feelings in ways not involving food.

Self-Esteem Eaters: Take the suggested steps to increase my feelings of self-worth.

Stress Eaters: Either lower my stress level or use stress
management tools other than food.

Snowball Effect Eaters: Be especially aware of my portion sizes.

All Yo-Yoers: Really believe in myself, and know that
I *can* lose the weight.

Regularly engage in my exercise program.

Other: _____

_____

Signed: _____   *Dated:* _____

Witness: _____   *Dated:* _____

port. You accidentally get off on the wrong freeway
exit. At that point, you don't just keep driving down
the wrong road, do you? No! As soon as you realize the
mistake you've made, you just get right back on the
freeway until you find the correct exit ramp.

Well, that's exactly how it is with your Yo-Yo Syndrome Diet, too. If you do—for any reason—find
yourself overeating, follow the suggestions below to
immediately get yourself back on the "freeway" toward
your destination. Don't keep driving on the wrong road
of an eating binge.

Here are ways to get back on your Diet should you
slip, overeat or binge:

- Call a friend who is also on the Yo-Yo Syndrome
  Diet. Talk with this person about your eating, and
  ask for emotional support as you get back on your
  Diet.
- Go to an Overeaters Anonymous meeting. While
  you are there, it's important that you talk about
  your slip even though it may be frightening, hu-
  miliating or humbling. After you talk about it,
  you'll feel renewed commitment to your Diet.
- Reread this book for additional reinforcement and
  support.
- Destroy any binge foods you have in your house,
  office or car. Don't wait to "give them away to a
  neighbor"—get rid of them now.

Although I don't wish a slip on *anybody,* I do want to
acknowledge that sometimes it is the best thing that can

happen to someone. Let me explain. I was seeing a new patient, Brian, because his mother Debra had done well on the Yo-Yo Syndrome Diet and she knew that her son needed this particular brand of help as well.

Brian, a 22-year-old college student, came reluctantly into therapy. He knew he wanted help with his excess weight, but he wasn't sure how a psychotherapist was going to be able to help him. Still, he kept reminding himself how much weight his mother had lost on my program. As I explained the concept of binge foods to Brian, he immediately told me that he knew his were salty junk foods. When I told him then about abstinence as a way of preventing eating binges, I could see that Brian didn't quite buy my theory. He signed the Yo-Yo Syndrome Diet Contract anyway, and for the next month he stayed away from salty junk foods completely. He even lost 11 pounds in the process!

Then Brian had to go out of state for one of his college courses. While he was away from all the reminders of his Yo-Yo Syndrome Diet, he ate his binge food, starting with one bag of potato chips. With this, Brian went into a full-blown eating binge that lasted until he returned home two months later and made an appointment to come see me.

When I saw Brian, I knew he was now convinced he was a Binge Eater. He had experienced firsthand an eating binge triggered by one bite of his binge food, and since he had gained knowledge and insight about his Yo-Yo Syndrome, he knew exactly what he had to do. Brian, because of his slip, had completely accepted that he needed to abstain from his binge food forever, a day at a time.

And that's why slips can sometimes be beneficial. Before his slip, Brian was staying away from salty junk food purely to please me and his mother. Following his eating binge, however, Brian's motivation became purely internal—he was abstaining because he was absolutely sure there was no such thing as just one bite. This internal motivation makes all the difference in the Yo-Yo Syndrome Diet.

Struggling with Those Last Few Pounds

Most of us know the struggle of losing those final five to ten pounds before reaching goal weight. Up until that point, your weight has come off with relative ease; now you come to a grinding halt as you get closer and closer to your final destination. At this point, you may become frustrated and overwhelmed. Some people even decide to stay at the weight they've landed at, making that their goal weight. And that's okay, as long as you are happy at the weight you've reached. If you're satisfied with the weight your body naturally veers toward, then that's what counts.

If, however, you really do want to shave off those extra few pounds, then you owe it to yourself to go for it. Here are some tips which can help push you over the weight edge and onto your goal weight:

- Intensify your exercise program. If you're now exercising four days a week, you may need to work out five days for a while to get those last stubborn pounds off. If you're in the beginner's aerobics class, you may need to try the next level of difficulty. If you're walking half a mile a day, try one mile instead for a while.

- Focus on staying on your Diet today and congratulate yourself on each pound that you lose. In other words, don't look at your weight loss negatively ("Oh my gosh, I've only lost sixteen pounds since I started this diet. I've got over ten more pounds to lose! I'll never get there.") because you'll end up discouraged and overwhelmed. Instead, focus on one pound at a time. Take a positive approach ("Great! I've lost two pounds since Wednesday. Now I'll focus on losing two more pounds.") and you'll find your motivation stays high and your progress and weight loss on the Yo-Yo Syndrome Diet will be satisfying.

- Have a pair of jeans on hand that will fit you once you reach your goal weight. Try them on every morning to serve as a reminder that *you're not quite there yet* (this will help you resist temptations throughout the day), and help you see any progress you are making in your weight-loss process. Maybe the jeans don't zip up all the way today, but at least they fit a little better than they did last week!

- Remember to picture yourself at your goal weight so that your behavior matches your picture. How do thin people eat? Most of us imagine thin people eating very slowly and kind of picking at their food. Talking more than eating. And putting their eating utensils down all the time. If you can picture yourself as a thin person, then you'll naturally start to mimic these slimming behaviors yourself.

- Increase your water intake. Barring health restrictions (such as some cardiovascular disorders, which your doctor should advise you about), you can never drink too much water! Water also has an amazing way of getting people off of weight plateaus. If you're drinking one-half gallon a day now, then try drinking one gallon instead and see if that doesn't budge the scale for you. The side benefits of a clearer complexion, decreased appetite and all the exercise of running to the bathroom also make drinking plenty of water a good idea.

- Cut out red meats entirely until you reach your goal weight. I've had clients whose weight wouldn't budge until they took this step and substituted fish and chicken for beef and pork. If you are on a plateau, maybe you should try this, too.

- Some Yo-Yo Syndrome sufferers, who have particularly slow metabolisms due to their years of countless diets, may need to cut their calorie count below the 1200 (1500 for men) recommended in the Yo-Yo Syndrome Diet. To do this, simply cut out one of your snacks (but never skip a meal to cut calories).

- Refuse to give up! No matter how frustrating a weight plateau is, don't let it get the best of you.

Besides, it would be illogical to gain all the weight back just because you're momentarily frustrated.

If you follow the steps of the Yo-Yo Syndrome Diet, the weight will come off. You may be used to those fad diets that rapidly took the pounds off, and it's important to remember that this diet is different in that weight loss will be a little slower. Fast diets just don't result in permanent weight losses or permanent changes in eating behavior in the way that balanced, realistic and slower diets do.

Maintaining Your Loss

You've done it! You've reached your goal weight and you look and feel fantastic! Even though you've probably been thin like this before, this time you're going to *stay* thin.

I remember the last time I lost all my excess weight. I was happy, of course, but I also expected to start putting all the weight back on again. I was so accustomed to gaining weight immediately after losing it that it actually felt odd to keep the weight off. Just as your equilibrium makes you feel as though you're still swaying in the waves after stepping off a rocking boat onto firm ground, I felt a strong momentum to keep going with my past pattern of gaining and losing, losing and gaining.

But I also was determined to try to keep it off this

time. I say "try" because, since I'd never experienced staying thin, I wasn't exactly sure I was capable of it. My only hope, I knew, was to keep taking my diet one day at a time. And I used all of the tips that are outlined in this book; believe me, I needed all the help I could get.

Once you have reached your goal weight, there are several steps to take:

1. *Go back to measuring your food if you have stopped.* This is important because you're going to be increasing your portions in small increments (see #3, below).

2. *Keep weighing yourself and looking at yourself in the mirror daily.* If, at any time during your Yo-Yo Syndrome Maintenance Diet, your weight increases by two or more pounds, *don't ignore it!* Figure out immediately the source of the extra poundage and nip this weight gain in the bud before it climbs into another upward yo-yo.

Ask yourself the following questions:

- "Did I gain the weight from eating at a restaurant last evening?" If so, then you probably either had too big a meal or food that was high in sodium (such as the MSG used at Oriental restaurants). Plan to avoid that restaurant, eat a much smaller meal there the next time, or ask that the food be prepared without salt or MSG.
- "Did I gain the weight from making my portions too big yesterday?" If so, then reread and review Step #1 according to your Yo-Yo Syndrome Style.

It's important to change your old habits of eating before this two-pound weight gain slips into a huge weight gain!

- "Did I gain the weight from eating foods that aren't on the Yo-Yo Syndrome Diet?" Perhaps you're using whole milk instead of skim, or are eating red meats more than once a week. If this is the case, reread Chapters 7 and 8 and plan on going back on the Yo-Yo Syndrome Diet for at least one week. After the two pounds are off again, then return to the Maintenance Diet (described in #3, below).

- "Did I gain the weight from not exercising enough?" If you've let your fitness program slip, you'll be burning calories at a slower rate. Reread Chapter 9 and recommit yourself to physical fitness.

- "Did I gain the weight from skipping meals?" As discussed in Chapter 7, if you skip a meal, your body won't burn calories efficiently and you're likely to overeat at the following meal. If you're doing "creative dieting" at all, reread Chapter 7.

- "Did I gain the weight from eating my binge food?" Binge Eaters who eat their binge food will find their eating becomes out of control. For this very important reason, it's vital for Binge Eaters to adhere to Step #3 of their Yo-Yo Syndrome Diet: Abstain from your binge food.

- "Did I gain the weight from having too large a snack?" Is your after-dinner snack an endless feast of finger foods? If so, then you may be someone who can't snack (see Chapter 7). Some people are just unable to stop eating after they have a snack. These folks need to have their snacks immediately after lunch and dinner, then brush their teeth and stick to non-caloric fluids and sugarless gum until it's time for their next meal.

- "Did I gain the weight from retaining water?" If you're not drinking eight glasses of water a day, chances are your weight gain is from fluid retention. This is especially true if you're eating foods high in sodium or are drinking more than two diet colas a day. It's important to keep your water intake high in order to flush out excess salt and water.

3. *Begin Your Yo-Yo Syndrome Maintenance Diet.* The key to the success of the Maintenance Diet is that it slowly adds food back to your meals and gives you time to see how each addition affects your weight. Everyone's metabolism, after all, is different and burns calories at a different rate. Those of us who have dieted over and over have extremely slow metabolisms, while people who've dieted only once or twice burn calories quicker. Men tend to have more efficient metabolisms than women, and heavier people tend to lose weight quicker than those closer to their goal weights. In addition, exercise speeds up metabolism.

Since everyone is so different, only you will know how much food you can eat and still successfully maintain your weight loss. I'd like to see you stay at your goal weight, with a fluctuation of plus or minus two pounds. In other words, if your goal weight is 120 pounds, you should never veer below 118 or above 122. If you do, then reread and recommit yourself to the steps of the Yo-Yo Syndrome Diet.

It's almost impossible to stay at exactly the same weight without some minor fluctuations, usually brought on by fluid retention (especially during menstrual cycles). This is the same as when you drive your car down a perfectly straight road—you tend to move the steering wheel ever so slightly.

What we want to avoid—at all costs—are the sharp veers that would send you off the road and into a ditch. Memorize this: No More Yo-Yoing!

YO-YO SYNDROME MAINTENANCE DIET

Addition #1—First month following attainment of goal weight: *Add one meat serving to your daily diet.*

You can add this to any one meal or have an extra portion with your dinner. Keep in mind that you still need to limit red meat consumption to once a week or less.

If after one month you are still at your goal weight (plus or minus two pounds), then go on to the next maintenance addition. If you have gained over two pounds, then remove the meat addition from your daily diet and stay with the original Yo-Yo Syndrome Diet.

Addition #2—Second month following attainment and maintenance of goal weight: *Add a snack, and have it after breakfast.*

Between breakfast and lunch, have a late-morning snack from the list given in Chapter 7. If this results in a weight gain of over two pounds at the end of one month, then delete this snack and use only Addition #1 above. If, however, you still haven't gained weight (beyond the two-pound fluctuation maximum), after one month of eating both the additional serving of meat and this late-morning snack, go on to Addition #3 below.

Addition #3—Third month following attainment and maintenance of goal weight: *Add one starch serving to your lunch.*

This can mean an extra serving of rice, bread, potatoes or beans at lunchtime. And again, if after one month you've gained weight, then delete this addition. If you've still maintained your great new shape, then go on to Addition #4.

Addition #4—Fourth month following attainment and maintenance of goal weight: *Add one starch serving to your dinner.*

If this doesn't result in a weight gain after one month, then go on to Addition #5. If it does, then return to Addition #3.

Addition #5—Fifth month following attainment and maintenance of goal weight: *Double the portion size of your mid-afternoon snack.*

Instead of choosing one item from the snack list outlined in Chapter 7, choose two to have simultaneously between lunch and dinner. As with the other Additions, your weight after one month will determine whether you should remove this extra snack or keep it in your diet.

Few people could add more calories than these five additions without gaining weight, but again, it's up to you to keep on top of the relationship between what the scale says and what you put into your mouth. If you ever find yourself gaining more than two pounds, then immediately cut back your Additions until the extra poundage comes off.

You Can Do It!

No matter what you've been told in the past, no matter what negative beliefs you've held about yourself, you really can have the body you want. It doesn't matter how old you are, how much money you do or don't have, how many years you went to school, or anything else—you can lose weight now and keep it off for good!

Keep in mind that *every time* you pick up your fork or spoon, you are engaged in the process of making a choice. You are choosing, at that moment, what size body to have. If you overeat or indulge in fattening foods, your body will be heavy. If you eat right, according to the Yo-Yo Syndrome Diet, your body will remain slim. That choice and responsibility lie solely with you.

Just because you want a certain food, just because you'd love to have a second helping, doesn't mean you have to eat it. You probably have other impulses (like fantasizing about that good-looking person) that you'd never follow through on. Put eating in the same category and begin to distinguish between a desire for something, and a decision to carry it through. They are entirely different processes.

Similarly, a hunger pang does not necessarily signal that it's time to eat. As discussed throughout this book, sometimes what feels like hunger is actually an emotion or stress in disguise. And it will take your stomach approximately a month to get used to the low-fat diet. Hunger pangs, to me, are a signal that my body's efficiently using up all its calories, so I look at them in a positive vein.

If you follow the steps outlined in this book, you'll never need to spend another dime on diet books, weight-loss clubs or other futile methods. Everything you need to lose weight is contained in these pages.

I can't tell you what a difference the Yo-Yo Syndrome Diet has made in my life! How good it feels:

To wear the same size jeans in January as in July.

To be able to wear a swimsuit out in public and not feel the need to wear a bath towel around my hips.

To wear shorts even before I have a tan on my legs.

To have fun wearing the newest fashions, no matter how skimpy they are.

To try on clothes and like the way they look on me in the dressing room mirror.

To receive admiring glances from men.

To have others compliment me on my figure.

To hear my husband continually compliment me on the way I look.

To hear my sons tell me I look pretty.

But beyond all these external extras, the main benefits I've received from the Yo-Yo Syndrome Diet are a tremendous amount of self-respect, confidence and self-love. This is the main difference between this and your average diet plan—I know, because I've been thin many times in the past, but was never before able to enjoy it because I didn't like myself very much.

Besides helping me lose weight, the Yo-Yo Syndrome Diet has taught me how to be good to myself. I learned that I could tailor my life so that I could be happy! And that knowledge gave me the courage to take risks so that my real life could match the one I'd always dreamed of. I set occupational, educational, financial, spiritual, physical and emotional goals for myself. I put those goals on my affirmations tape (see Chapter 4) and listened to them daily. And because of my subsequently high level of self-esteem and my belief in myself, I was able to achieve every one of my goals.

I don't want to sound as if I'm bragging, because I'm not. What I want you to know, though, is that I'm no different from you in any way. It wasn't that many years ago when I was 55 pounds overweight, had no college education, worked at a minimum-wage job that I despised and could barely pay my bills—and my future seemed as bleak as my life was then.

At that time, I was really down on myself. I felt fat, ugly and unlovable. My only source of comfort seemed to come from a carton of chocolate ice cream. And even though I hated my bulging thighs that scraped together as I walked, I didn't know I had any other option. I didn't know there was any better way to live. Happiness, I believed, was a myth perpetuated by TV soap operas. Other people were thin. Other people had nice houses and cars. I just didn't think it was in my cards to have a nice life.

Thank God I know differently today! Thank God I escaped from that living hell!

Today, every day is a celebration with lots of smiles and feelings of gratitude for all the emotional and physical riches that have come my way. Sure, it has meant a lot of work and painful introspection during the process when I was getting to know myself. Going to college all those years and working with my patients was at times a struggle. And there were moments when I would have killed for chocolate ice cream.

But I can assure you, as one who has been on both sides of the fence, that the life I lead today—as a thin person who is living the dream she orchestrated for herself—tastes a million times better than any scoop of ice cream I ever had!

DOREEN VIRTUE is a psychotherapist who specializes in treating Yo-Yo Syndrome sufferers. She founded and directs an eating-disorder and weight-loss clinic in southern California and regularly lectures on the Yo-Yo Syndrome.

You have just finished reading
one of the first books published
by Harper Paperbacks!

Please continue to look for
the sign of the 'H', below.

It will appear on many fiction
and non-fiction books, from
literary classics to dazzling
international bestsellers.

And it will always stand for a
great reading experience and a
well-made book.

Harper Paperbacks
10 East 53rd St.
New York, NY 10022